T0136767

Psychopathology: An Empathic Representational Approach

Psychopathology

An Empathic Representational Approach

An Integration of Phenomenology and
Cognitive Neuroscience

Eric Yu Hai Chen

HKU
PRESS
香港大學出版社

Hong Kong University Press
The University of Hong Kong
Pokfulam Road
Hong Kong
https://hkupress.hku.hk

© 2022 Hong Kong University Press

ISBN 978-988-8754-25-0 (*Hardback*)

British Library Cataloguing-in-Publication Data
A catalogue record for this book is available from the British Library.

10 9 8 7 6 5 4 3 2 1

Printed and bound by J&S Printing Co., Ltd. in Hong Kong, China

Contents

Detailed Analyses of Contents

Figures

Foreword

Since its coinage in 1847, the term 'psychopathology' has accrued so many meanings that currently it is little more than a portmanteau. By the end of the previous century, it had about 14 meanings;[1] others have been added since. Polysemic terms have, of course, a role in literature but they may not be particularly useful in medicine.

So, in order for psychopathology to play a role in the complex business of psychiatry, it needs to be restructured and provided with an adequate epistemological basis. Professor Chen's book is an effort in this direction.

Origins of Psychopathology

In his 1845 book, *Lehrbuch der ärztliche Seelenkunde*,[2] Feuchtersleben stated that *Psychopathologie* (p. 69) had not yet gained sufficient knowledge about the mechanisms of madness. In all likelihood, the author wanted for alienism something similar to the new discipline of *Physio-pathologie*, that is, the study of abnormal function in disease. His English translators decided, for some unclear reason, to delete the hyphen.[3] Thus, the term 'psychopathology' (p. 70) was introduced into the English language.

But this only explains the origin of the word. There was not yet content for the putative concept it named given that Feuchtersleben's hope could not be achieved. Psychopathology reappeared in the second half of the nineteenth century, in the work of Emminghaus,[4] Störring,[5] Marie,[6] and others but only to name the collection of descriptions of mental symptoms, that is, an activity known before as semiology (*séméïologie générale*).[7]

---

1. Ionescu, S. (1991). *Quatorze approaches de la psychopathologie*. Nathan.
2. Feuchtersleben, E. (1845). *Lehrbuch der ärztliche Seelenkunde*. Carl Gerold.
3. Feuchtersleben, E. (1847). *Principles of medical psychology* (H. E. Lloyd & B. G. Babington, Trans.). Sydenham Society.
4. Emminghaus, H. (1878). *Allgemeine Psychopathologie zur Einführung in das Studium der Geistesstörungen*. Vogel.
5. Störring, G. (1900). *Vorlesungen über Psychopathologie*. Wilhem Engelmann.
6. Marie, A. (Ed.). (1912). *Traité International de Psychopathologie Pathologique. Tome Deuxième: Psychopathologie Clinique*. Alcan.
7. Double, F. J. (1811). *Séméïologie générale, ou traité des signes et de leur valeur dans les maladies* (3 Vols.). Croullebois.

Semiology did not disappear altogether for the historian finds it in the great text-books by Morselli and Chaslin.[8] But the word 'psychopathology' won the day and started to become fashionable at the beginning of the twentieth century. This is the reason why, through Professor Karl Wilmanns,[9] Ferdinand Springer invited the young Karl Jaspers to write *Allgemeine Psychopathologie*.[10]

It can be concluded that in the nineteenth century, psychopathology was far closer to semiology than to physiopathology. Most alienists settled on the view that the new discipline was about the capture and description of mental symptoms. Indeed, during the period aetiological speculation is only to be found in textbooks of psychiatry.

Influences on Psychopathology

All this was to change after two important late-nineteenth-century developments: the growth of clinical psychology and the emergence of psychoanalysis.

As empirical disciplines, psychology and later clinical psychology developed during the second half of the nineteenth century. They soon took charge of the naming and classification of mental functions,[11] and sought to impose these names upon psychopathology. Some of these functions had already been adopted by psychiatrists influenced by Kant and faculty psychology.[12] Other high-level categories, for example, personality, were new and research started to identify how their 'dysfunction' could be clinically expressed.[13] Lastly, first-wave clinical psychologists such as Janet, Ribot, and Piéron started to add explanations to the description of mental symptoms.[14] This trend was continued into the twentieth century, for example, in the work of behaviourists,[15] Eysenck,[16] and more recently cognitive psychologists.

The advent of psychoanalysis was also important. Under its aegis psychopathology became far more than a semiology, and description of mental symptoms gave way to complex interpretations.[17] After the 1910s, this change can increasingly be seen in

8.   Morselli, E. (1885). *Manuale di Semejotica delle Malattie Mentali*. 2 vols. Vallardi; Chaslin, Ph. (1912). *Éléments de sémiologie et clinique mentales*. Asselin et Houzeau.
9.   Mundt, C. H., Hoffmann, K., & Wilmanns, J. (2011). Karl Wilmanns' theoretische Ansätze und klinische Praxis. *Nervenarzt, 82*, 79–89.
10. Jaspers, K. (1977). *Philosophische Autobiographie* (pp. 22–23). R. Piper; Jaspers, K. (1913). *Allgemeine psychopathologie*. Springer.
11. Danziger, K. (1997). *Naming the mind*. Sage.
12. Hilgard, E. R. (1980). The trilogy of mind cognition, affection and conation. *Journal of the History of the Behavioral Sciences, 16*, 107–117; Brooks, G. P. (1976). The faculty psychology of Thomas Reid. *Journal of the History of the Behavioral Sciences, 12*, 65–77; Albrecht, F. M. (1970). A re-appraisal of faculty psychology. *Journal of the History of Behavioural Science, 6*, 36–40.
13. Berrios, G. E. (1993). European views on personality disorders: A conceptual history. *Comprehensive Psychiatry, 34*, 14–30.
14. Nicolas, S. (2002). *Histoire de la psychologie française. Naissance d'un nouvelle science*. In Press Éditions.
15. Tryon, W. W., Ferster, C. B., & Franks, C. M. (1980). On the role of behaviourism in clinical psychology. *The Pavlovian Journal of Biological Science, 15*, 12–20.
16. Eysenck, H. J. (Ed.). (1958). *Handbook of abnormal psychology: An experimental approach*. Pitman.
17. Masling, J. M., & Bornstein, R. F. (Eds.). (1994). *Psychoanalytic perspectives on psychopathology*. APA Books.

'psychopathology' books.[18] Lastly, the lasting impact of psychoanalysis is one of the explanations for why in the USA the word 'psychopathology' is used as almost tantamount to 'psychiatry'.[19]

Epistemological Worth of Psychopathology

The above historical vicissitudes explain the polysemy of psychopathology but say little about its clinical usefulness, that is, the role that a description of mental symptoms plays in the management of sufferers. This is because usefulness is a function of the epistemological power of psychopathology, that is, of its capacity to obtain 'knowledge'.

'Knowledge' in this context means the finding of stable, negotiated narratives (which are simultaneously cognitive, emotional, aesthetic, and rhetorical) with predictive power and the capacity to generate meaningful and efficient therapies. If this is not achieved, then psychopathology becomes an exercise in futility.

Efforts to assess the epistemological power of psychopathology started during the nineteenth century. *Ab initio*, these concentrated on evaluating the quality of medical examination and conceptually relied on notions such as the clinical eye and introspection.[20]

When during the early twentieth century the epistemology of introspection came under attack from psychology,[21] psychoanalysis,[22] and philosophy,[23] 'interpretations' of mental symptoms started to be preferred to detailed descriptions.

In 1913, Jaspers came to the rescue by claiming 'phenomenology' could provide a solid epistemological justification for psychopathology. By doing so he summoned in favour of clinical descriptivism the power of what, at the time, was a very popular philosophical movement.[24]

Things have changed little since. Within psychiatry there is the tacit agreement that descriptive psychopathology can be supported by some sort of undefined 'phenomenological' conceptualization. By parading Jaspers's 'foundationalism' in the first pages, most European texts of descriptive psychopathology avoid providing their own epistemological justification.

This also seems to be the case with the skeletal definitions of mental symptoms listed at the end of various DSM glossaries, which although parasitical upon the classical

---

18. Berrios, G. E. (1991). British psychopathology since the early 20th century. In G. E. Berrios & H. Freeman (Eds.), *150 years of British psychiatry* (pp. 232–244). Gaskell.

19. Sutker, P. B., & Adams, H. E. (2002). *Comprehensive handbook of psychopathology* (3rd ed.). Kluwer; Helzer, J. E., & Hudziak, J. J. (Eds.). (2002). *Defining psychopathology in the 21st century.* American Psychopathological Association.

20. Boring, E. G. (1953). A history of introspection. *Psychological Bulletin, 50,* 169–189.

21. Danziger, K. (1980). The history of introspection reconsidered. *Journal of the History of the Behavioral Sciences, 16,* 241–262.

22. Perron, R. (2005). Introspection. In A. Mijolla (Ed.), *International dictionary of psychoanalysis* (p. 871). Gale.

23. Lyons, W. (1986). *The disappearance of introspection.* MIT Press.

24. Berrios, G. E. (1992). Phenomenology, psychopathology and Jaspers: A conceptual history. *History of Psychiatry, 3,* 303–327.

European descriptions want to give the impression that the definitions are written in stone and now lie outside time.

The Statistical Treatment of Psychopathology

Three ongoing fashions seem to be based on the current, unfounded belief that the definitions of mental symptoms have come to stay. One concerns the proliferation of rating instruments and scales. Once used to evaluate severity, the fashion now is to consider them as solid diagnostic tools. To many, rating scales are imbued with the special power of transforming categorical quality into a quantifiable dimension.[25] And to others this type of quantification may even bestow some form of perpetual 'objectivity' upon the data. This is why rating scales are applied mechanically, for example, via the internet. The fact that all the original scale-makers believed that dialogical context was essential to modulate item scores does not seem to worry current users.[26]

The second fashion concerns the view that psychopathology needs 'resharpening'. It is implied that psychopathology was once a 'precision tool' and it, for some reason, has lost its edge.[27] The sharpening in question can be achieved by linking the narratives of psychopathology to the hard neurosciences. Inspired by real science, psychopathology may play a role in the new 'precision psychiatry'.

Others want to interrogate psychopathology the hard way. Large data sets should be subjected to high-power statistical analysis. Such treatment should force the data of psychopathology to divulge patterns and other information that have been hiding for centuries. It is predicted that deep down psychopathology is actually structured in hierarchical dimensions, super-spectra, spectra, sub-factors, syndromes, components, symptoms, and so forth.[28] Once these hidden structures have been found, it is less clear how they should relate to patients in the clinic.

Close to the above is the older proposal of the Research Domain Criteria (RDoC),[29] which assume that subjecting to statistical analysis combinations of all manner of variables (psychopathological, social, neuroscientific, etc.), patterns, and structures could emerge, which could be recognized as new mental disorders.

In general, this approach seems to assume that the information obtained in the mental state examination, just like platonic ideas, has eternal ontology and that once

25. Berrios, G. E., & Marková, I. S. (2013). Is the concept of 'dimension' applicable to psychiatric objects? *World Psychiatry, 12,* 76–78.
26. Berrios, G. E., & Bulbena-Villarasa, A. (1990). The Hamilton Depression Scale and the numerical description of the symptoms of depression. In P. Bech & A. Coppen (Eds.), *The Hamilton Scales* (pp. 80–92). Springer.
27. Schultze-Lutter, F., Schmidt, S. J., & Theodoridou, A. (2018). Psychopathology: A precision tool in need of resharpening. *Frontiers in Psychiatry, 9,* 1–6.
28. Lahey, B. B., Moore, T. M., Kaczkurkin, A. N., & Zald, D. H. (2021). Hierarchical models of psychopathology: Empirical support, implications, and remaining issues. *World Psychiatry, 20,* 57–63.
29. Cuthbert, B. N., & Kozak, M. J. (2013). Constructing constructs for psychopathology: The NIMH research domain criteria. *Journal of Abnormal Psychology, 122,* 928–937.

saved in a hard disk it will keep forever. This approach also disregards contextual information which is known to provide symptom recognition with meaning.[30]

The interesting issue here is that some of the questions above have an empirical
answer. Before embarking in grandiose numerical exercises, workers should ask what
the epistemological shelf life of their data is, even within the same patient. For example,
are the 'hallucinations' found in the first episode the same clinical phenomenon (in
both psychological and neuroscientific terms) as the 'hallucinations' found twenty
years later?

Whither Psychopathology?

Books like Professor Chen's rekindle a much-needed dialogue about psychopathology,
its meaning, and its future. In this regard, I want to consider just three options.

One is for psychopathology to return to its original calling and become a sort
of 'physiopathology' of mental symptoms, that is, a set of empirical accounts of how
mental symptoms are actually constructed.

To achieve this aim, psychopathologists will have to abandon their enthralment
to 'brainhood',[31] that is, the view that madness must only be about the brain. When at
the beginning of the nineteenth century alienism began to be constructed, the stomach
was very much in running as a site for madness.[32] For almost two centuries 'brainhood'
has reigned supreme. It would seem that of late the good old digestive system is being
reconsidered.[33]

The second option for psychopathology is to remain at a descriptive level and try
to reinforce its epistemological value by re-examining introspection,[34] by reaffirming
its dialogical and contextual basis and developing some pride in its narrative quality.[35]
It will have to show that (1) the type of knowledge obtained in the clinical dialogue is
qualitative, broader, and deeper than mere cognitive information; (2) statistical treatment of the information obtained attenuates or deletes important nuances hidden in
the descriptions; and (3) there are no hidden patterns in large conglomerations of data
for they do not originate from a closed platonic universe; on the contrary, they exhibit
the same volatility as the rest of the cultural objects.

The third option for psychopathology is just to curl up in the corner of a historical library and die. In this Brave New World, all psychiatric diagnosis will be done by

30. Berrios, G. E., & Chen, E. Y. H. (1993). Recognizing psychiatric symptoms: Relevance to the diagnostic
    process. *British Journal of Psychiatry, 163*, 308–314.
31. Vidal, F., & Ortega, F. (2017). *Being brains: Making the cerebral subject*. Fordham University Press.
32. Broussais, F. J. V. (1828). *De L'Irritation et de la Folie*. Delaunay.
33. Severance, E. G., Prandovszky, E., Castiglione, J., & Yolken, R. H. (2015). Gastroenterology issues in schizo-
    phrenia: Why the gut matters. *Current Psychiatry Reports, 17*, 27–43.
34. Berrios, G. E., & Marková, I. S. (2015). Towards a new epistemology of psychiatry. In L. J. Kirmayer,
    R. Lemelson, & C. Cummings (Eds.), *Revisioning psychiatry: Cultural phenomenology, critical neuroscience and
    global mental health* (pp. 41–64). Cambridge University Press.
35. Marková, I. S., & Berrios, G. E. (2009). The epistemology of mental symptoms. *Psychopathology, 42*, 343–349;
    Marková, I. S., & Berrios, G. E. (2012). The epistemology of psychiatry. *Psychopathology, 45*, 220–227.

markers, and precision psychiatry will find the exact cure. Psychopathology may even be made to survive as a sort of conversational piece, a nicety that courteous psychiatrists (or computers) will want to exchange with sufferers (or carriers or disease) whilst the real stuff is going on.

Professor Chen and His Book

It is a pleasure to see that Professor Chen, once upon a time an active member of the Cambridge Psychopathology Group,[36] remains active in this field and has now decided to throw his hat into the ring. His book deserves the most attentive of readings. I wish it every success. Indeed, the future of psychopathology may partly depend upon the kind of stir it should produce.

Professor German E. Berrios
University of Cambridge, 2021

---

36. Marková, I. S., & Chen, E. Y. H. (Eds.). (2020). *Rethinking Psychopathology: Creative Convergences*. Springer.

Preface

This book is an in-depth exploration of psychopathology as subjective experiences that reflect underlying dysfunctions in the brain. Psychopathology is important because there are natural patterns in the disruptive experiences that may help us in arriving at a better understanding of the underlying conditions and hence better treatments.

Generations of clinicians and researchers have pondered upon how to distil the information contained in these subjective experiences. Access to subjective experience is a complex business and requires substantial skills, which is sometimes neglected in today's clinical practice. In our fast-paced world, it can be tempting to reduce psychopathological evaluations to simple processes such as checklists. Related to this is the reductionist optimism that measures such as brain scans may provide the required information instead. This hope turns out to be over-simplistic. An integrated approach is needed.

The richness of the emerging psychopathological information demands a reflection on the adequacy of our underlying model for human experiences. A more fit-for-purpose psychopathology framework may be critical in meeting the needs of modern psychiatry, for example, in early symptom and risk-states detection.

Descriptions of human subjective experiences involve skills and knowledge shared by a broad range of disciplines, including not only psychiatry, medicine, and psychology but also cognitive science, linguistics, ethnography, phenomenology, computational science and neuroscience. Psychopathology stands to benefit from harvesting the cross-fertilization of these fields, bringing together new insights, paving the way for enriching our understanding.

This exploration cannot be separated from the ongoing clinical, research, and teaching activities, which span more than a decade, during the active preparation of this work. Lively discussions with colleagues in different settings provide the background for this work.

This work serves as a platform to bring these dialogues to a wider range of clinicians, researchers, and students of psychopathology. It should also be of interest to those exploring related aspects of human experiences. In using this work, it is advisable to allow oneself sufficient time for an active interaction with the various ideas, to ponder and reflect upon them. Many of the topics can be fruitfully explored in group discussions.

It is becoming increasingly clear that contemporary psychopathology may have to deal with a 'moving target', with the realization that distress of the human mind can no longer be seen as a static object. The modern age has brought accelerating changes in the way people experience life. Studying this complex subject requires incorporating a capacity for embracing future changes. To this end, it is particularly important to build a foundation with sufficient breadth and depth to allow for timely responses to the ever-changing human experiences today.

Acknowledgements

In a book aspiring to cover such an extensive aspect of the human condition, it is essential to be able to have serious discussions with a group of people who can offer diverse perspectives from the heights of their respective fields. I am grateful that I have had the privilege to count on German Berrios, Robert Miller, Carver Yu, Ivana Marková, Georg Northoff, and Michael Wong to go through earlier versions of the manuscript. German mentored me into the challenging field of psychopathology, encouraged me to apply contemporary knowledge creatively to the field, and revealed to me the relevance of an historical approach to the subject. He is never more than a call away when I need a discussion. Robert, with the many refreshing discussions, uniquely brings his deep neuroscience insight and first-person reflections into the work. Carver critically evaluated the work with his profound knowledge in philosophical theology and deep passion for the human condition based on long years of pastoral work. Ivana provided painstaking and profound comments from the perspective of a clinician philosopher. Georg provided his comments as both a neuroimaging researcher and a philosopher. Michael reviewed the manuscript several times from end to end, from the hermeneutics and the clinician perspective. Together their generous comments and deep discussions have prompted me to further develop selected parts of the work, as well as to address some potentially difficult areas with further explorations and clarifications.

I would also like to thank Peter McKenna, Byron Good, Brita Elvevåg, Bill Honer, Peter Falkai, Pat McGorry, and Peter Jones. They are long-standing friends and colleagues in different parts of the world. Their works formed the clinical and research background upon which the psychopathological questions for this work are situated. Peter McKenna introduced me to the importance of serious cognitive investigations of language processes. Byron initiated me into the world of ethnography and anthropology, with their unique relevance to psychopathology. Brita brought her refreshing perspectives from cognitive neuroscience and computational linguistics. Regular reflective discussions with Bill and Peter Falkai have provided impetus to attempt new angles for psychiatry. Pat and Peter Jones have seeded the field of early intervention, with renewed awareness of the need for good psychopathological information.

A special thanks is due for my colleagues Stephanie Wong, Ivy Lau, Gloria Wong, Sherry Chan, Christy Hui, and Yi Nam Suen, who participated in many rich discussions arising from topics in this book. Steph's discussions have always been incisive and brings one back to basic principles; Ivy, with her steadfast curiosity, has been a prototype for the psychopathologist for whom this book is written; and Gloria, with her insatiable appetite for good ideas, together with Sherry, Christy, and Yi Nam, has over the years undertaken the difficult tasks of elevating some of the ideas into empirical paradigms.

This book would not have been completed without the steadfast assistance of Fiona Cheung, Jessica Fung, and Melody Xu, as well as the editorial team at Hong Kong University Press, in their painstaking efforts in working with the revisions, references, and figures and ensuring consistency in the format of the work through its different stages.

Finally, I thank my wife Linda and my daughters, Heidi and Dorothy, for putting up with my far-away thoughts from time to time throughout the long period of preparation for this work. Without their unquestioning support, it would have been hard to bring this work into fruition.

Introduction

An Empathic Representational Approach to Psychopathology: Integration of Phenomenology and Cognitive Neuroscience

Psychopathology is concerned with the study of experiences that are manifestations of disruptions to the healthy functioning of the mind (Berrios, 1996; Jaspers, 1913/1963; Marková & Berrios, 1995, 2009). Mental symptoms are expressed in the subjective experiences of mankind. This domain of knowledge traverses the Natural Sciences and the Human Sciences and presents unique conceptualization challenges. A framework that facilitates integration between cognitive science, brain science, and phenomenology is essential for progress.

Systematic investigations of anomalous subjective experiences facilitate the understanding of mental conditions. Psychopathological information is essential to guide treatment, to estimate prognosis, and to facilitate early detection of disorders. Psychopathology has achieved some successes, but it has also met with significant challenges. It is likely that subjective experiences contain information about anomalous brain states. This information is conventionally accessed through the use of rating scales, with their inherent limitations. If psychopathological phenomena could be better observed and integrated with relevant knowledge domains, they may contribute to better prediction models to advance intervention efforts.

The methodology of psychopathology needs to be reviewed alongside progress in the studies of subjective phenomena as well as in brain and cognitive sciences. This work contributes towards this effort: to encourage a more refined treatment of psychopathology that rejects a simple mechanistic approach. It seeks adequate handling of human subjective experiences, respecting their uniqueness and complexity (Berrios, 1994), while at the same time reaching out to bridge insights from brain and cognitive studies.

Several existing accounts provide a conventional description of mental symptoms (e.g., Fish & Hamilton, 1985; Oyebode, 2015). This work explores new perspectives rather than compiling a list of mental symptoms. It examines some underlying frameworks in psychopathology, in order to identify new bridges between psychopathology and other emerging fields of knowledge. The current approach focuses on mental representations as keys for understanding the relationship between the mind and the information it handles. This perspective provides novel insight about the problems that can arise when there are failures in the operations of mental representations. We consider how these may be linked with symptoms as described in classical descriptive psychopathology, such as those summarized in Karl Jaspers's *General psychopathology* (1913/1963), which articulated a methodology for systematic investigations of anomalous experiences. The phenomenological approach was adopted for this purpose (e.g., Jaspers, 1912/1968, although for a critical discussion see Berrios, 1992). We aim to connect descriptive psychopathology with relevant emerging approaches that have become available since then. These include the fields of language and communication, cognitive processes, evolutionary biology, information science, and cultural processes. We build upon earlier explorations of the bridges between subjective experience and brain biology (e.g., Andrieu, 2006; Varela & Shear, 1999). These works initiated an emphasis on the active roles of the subjective mind amidst a predominantly reductionist neuroscience. They also suggested integrating phenomenological data (as first-person accounts of lived experiences) with measurements of brain activities (e.g., gamma oscillations) to varying degrees of success. The current account encompasses a broader conceptual approach that locates the actions of the mind in an 'information' domain. It is proposed that a key level of analysis in psychopathology could be at the level of mental representations. The objective is not to dwell on the details of neuroscience studies but to generate innovative ideas relevant to psychopathology. In the perusal of this goal, we shall try to be as specific as possible in describing mental representations through algorithms. We shall see that this approach does not lead to a 'reductionist explaining away' of phenomena, but instead it facilitates a better grasp of the complexity of various phenomena in the context of a holistic perspective of the human person. Along these explorations, we shall ponder upon new conceptual perspectives that are encountered. From these, we select useful ideas for applications in psychopathology. New ideas are considered to be useful when they address observations not previously accounted for, when they provide more parsimonious accounts than existing theories, when they provide integration between divergent perspectives, when they provide predictions not originally presupposed, and when they can be organized into a coherent framework. This work presents some of these ideas to clinicians and researchers.

We start the discussion with a review of the status of psychopathology as an empirical discipline (Chapter 1). This review highlights the need to address the unique nature of subjective human experience as a non-material, non-repeatable, but partially communicable domain. Psychopathology needs to address its non-material yet biologically based roots. The connection with brain function needs to be articulated at a useful level of analysis and not to be over-simplified in a coarse reductionist fashion. In Chapter 2, we explore information-handling functions of the brain from a biological, evolutionary, perspective. A reflection of the nature of 'information' in the brain is vital for psychopathology. Cognitive structures that hold information (i.e., mental representations) are considered as keys for connecting biology with psychopathology. Mental representations are proposed as basic building blocks for phenomenal experiences. We refer to mental representations as a variety of cognitive structures in an individual that *stand for* (*represent*) 'objects' or 'states of affairs' in the environment. They are presumed to be implemented by brain processes involving structures that allow data computation. Mental representations can be communicated between individuals. Low-level representations are involved in perceptual processes. High-level representations are dynamic, adaptive, and potentially autonomous. The notion of 'representations' has inherited multiple meanings. In this work, the term 'representation' is primarily used to refer to individualist, cognitive, 'mental representations' rather than in the sense of interactionist, communal, 'social representations'. The term 'mental representation' is used to refer both to the *structure* that can be filled with informational content at different times and to a particular *filled structure* representing a particular external object at a particular point in time.

The roles of 'mental representations' as information receptacles are introduced so that the reader can consider their relevance alongside the exploration of human experience from a phenomenological perspective. Phenomenology refers to an approach that emphasizes the importance of returning to the direct, raw subjective experience as a starting point in human knowing. In Chapter 3, we explore a phenomenological account of the core structure of human subjective experiences (i.e., what we can know about the subjective human experience as someone who directly accesses this experience from a first-person perspective).

This exercise identifies the essential, minimal, components of momentary experience, highlighting the features of temporality, relational nature, and agency. In Chapter 4, these essential components are extended to different experiential domains in the longitudinally unfolding human person. One crucial domain is the relationship with other people. In Chapter 5, the phenomena of relating to other people through empathic processes are explored. This leads to a discussion of the pivotal role of empathy in human experience. Out of the many different possible approaches to empathy, our exploration is influenced by the early phenomenological work articulated by Stein (1916/1970), consistent with our preference for a minimalist starting point in phenomenology. This approach is also coherent with a framework for conceptualizing the person in a holistic manner.

It is through empathy that the mind acquires the capacity for reflection upon itself, as well as the ability to explore the natural environment empirically. We shall see that it is also through empathy that it is possible to clarify psychopathological phenomena, through the alignment of representations between participants of a clinical dialogue (see Chapter 9). In Chapter 6, we return to a more advanced account of mental representations, now ready to be applied to various levels of subjective phenomena. Importantly, this account also facilitates an appreciation of the potential effects of rapid changes in the digital technological environment upon human experiences. We discuss how mental representations can be made as explicit as possible with the help of simple computational models. These models prepare for a consideration of how breakdowns in mental representation may underlie anomalous experiences (Chapter 7). Chapter 8 provides a discussion on how mental representation dysfunctions can account for a variety of anomalous experiences, suggesting novel conceptualizations of anomalous experiences according to the different modes of breakdown. In Chapter 9, we conclude with a pragmatic consideration of how empathy is used for the clarification of psychopathological processes, using the mental representation approach articulated in the earlier parts of this work. We look into the clinical dialogue as a method to access psychopathological signals. We consider how empathic processes are involved in communicating anomalous experiences. With these new insights, we end the exploration with an integrated approach to psychopathological assessments.

The term 'psychopathology' is used notwithstanding its stem '-pathology' being often used in medicine to suggest cellular disease mechanisms. However, 'psychopathology' has traditionally been used to refer to descriptive studies of mental symptoms. Acknowledging these caveats, we shall continue to use the term 'psychopathology' for the sake of continuity.

1

The Problem of Psychopathological Knowledge

1.1 Can We Really Approach Psychopathology Empirically?

Psychopathology is largely concerned with human subjective experience. We shall start with the question: to what extent can subjective experience be studied scientifically? This turns out to be a pivotal question on which the uniqueness of psychopathology hinges.

The essence of empirical investigations in the Natural Sciences has been summarized by Popper (1962). This involves repeated observations of phenomena in Nature, followed by the generation of hypotheses to account for the observations. Scientific theories enable predictions of future phenomena. These predictions are then tested. Theories that do not tally with empirical observation are refuted. Theories consistent with observations are supported (but not confirmed). Progresses are made along theories that have been consistently supported. When we apply this Natural Science approach to the study of subjective experience, we encounter challenges.

Objectification is a key process in the Natural Sciences. The target phenomenon has to be observed consistently by different observers on different occasions. Observations are expected to be *reproducible*. Subjective experiences are, however, not totally objectifiable. They contain 'meanings' unique to the individual. Moreover, individual experiences are not entirely reproducible, as individuals change continuously with the passage of time. As life experience accumulates, the 'me' yesterday is different from the 'me' today, and will be different from the 'me' tomorrow. Limits to objectification and reproducibility raise concerns about the simplistic adoption of Natural Science methods.

1.1.1 The gap between Natural Sciences and subjective experiences

In response to this, some thinkers would go as far as suggesting that there is an unbridgeable gap between the Natural Sciences and subjective phenomena. They suggest that the Natural Sciences and human experiences are two separate domains of knowledge. Consequently, it has been proposed that fundamentally different approaches should be utilized to investigate these two domains. For example, Weber (1922/1968) argued for the study of subjective phenomena through 'interpretive' means instead of 'empirical' means. He contended that an 'interpretive' approach would be more appropriate in the understanding of human experiences where individual intentions and meanings are involved (Dilthey, 1961; Weber, 1922/1968).

Pylyshyn (1984) suggested that human experiences could be viewed as the result of two different levels of brain-cognitive processes: The basic level of 'functional architecture' consists of the most basic operations of the brain (such as attention or memory). These processes are the 'building blocks' for more complex experiences. Intentions and meanings are handled at the higher, 'cognitively penetrable', level. It was proposed that processes that belong to the basic building blocks (i.e., 'functional architecture') are within the reach of the Natural Sciences, while those in the 'cognitively penetrable' level may require an interpretive approach.

1.1.2 Symptoms and signs in psychopathology

Within medicine, clinical observations are divided into symptoms and signs. Symptoms are subjective distresses (e.g., pain or dizziness) that people experience and communicate to clinicians. Signs are observations that the clinician made upon examination of the patient's body. Clinical observations are made systematically using a standardized method (e.g., examination of a mass in the abdomen). In examining clinical signs, the clinician treats the patient's body as a Natural Science object. However, in the examination of signs in the nervous system, the clinician often observes the behavioural *responses* of the patient in reaction to a standard stimulus (e.g., tendon reflexes). For observation of some nervous system functions, cognitive responses to standard stimuli are elicited (e.g., memory). Some functions are better observed in a spontaneous unstructured setting (e.g., prefrontal cortex functions, abnormalities in voluntary motor actions). When mental illnesses involve clinical signs, they are often best observed in a less-structured setting. Therefore, part of the clinical examination involves observing the spontaneous behaviour of the patient. This includes the behaviour of the patient in the clinical dialogue during which the experiences of the patient are also communicated. Thus, during the clinical dialogue, two fundamentally different processes proceed at the same time. Observation of dialogue behaviour belongs to the realms of the Natural Sciences. Communication of subjective experience as dialogue contents belongs to the realms of the Human Sciences.

1.1.3 Can positivist empiricism close the gap?

Recent approaches to the study of the mind have generally assumed an optimistic view that empirical methods can address most, if not all, subjective phenomena. Many of these approaches fail to acknowledge the difference in the subject matter (Natural Sciences objects usually have a material basis, have mass, and occupy space; subjective phenomena are non-material, have no mass, and do not occupy space). Some approaches impose Natural Science methods to the investigation of subjective experiences and, in the process, under-recognize their differences. One example is the use of rating scales to 'measure' subjective phenomena. Rating scales truncate contexts and standardize information in order to generate quantifiable data (e.g., an item on a rating scale such as 'I found it difficult to trust people' could be rated as 'high' in a certain context, say, after an actual experience of being cheated, but such contexts are often left out in rating scales). Often the numerical scores are treated as if they were data obtained by instrumental measurements. Such practices disregard the fundamental differences between material objects and subjective experience. If clinicians and researchers are unaware of their limitations, it is easy to over-interpret the numerical data.

Some researchers emphasize the importance of brain markers such as neuroimaging and electrophysiology, as they can be empirically studied with direct instrumental measurements. However, brain imaging cannot provide a full account of the subjective experience. We shall consider this question in the following sections.

1.1.4 The limits of brain markers in understanding subjective experiences

The possibility that brain states underlie subjective experiences is a widespread working assumption (Crick, 1994). For example, brain imaging has been used to identify brain systems associated with different *types of* mental activities. However, an important question is whether we can 'read off' subjective experiences from such data, even if we are capable of measuring all the data from every individual neuron and their connections in the brain. The crucial question hinges on whether meaning (or semantics), an essential component of experience, is represented in a uniform manner across individual brains (e.g., part of the multiple realizability problem, e.g., Borsboom et al., 2019). We ask whether for similar experiences the same physical brain structures are involved in different individuals, or whether similar experiences are instantiated by *functionally equivalent* sets of neurons (i.e., defined by their connection with other neurons in the individualized semantic net rather than by absolute anatomical locations; in other words, there is no absolute, external anatomical reference of individual neurons encoding specific meanings). There is no reason why structurally these networks cannot be represented by neurons located differently in different individuals (i.e., only relational connectivity needs to be preserved). For example, we know that after brain damage a new functionally equivalent network can regenerate at an alternative brain location (Wang et al., 2010). This sets a limit to the extent to which brain state data can specify subjective experiences. If this were the case, even if we can specify the activities of every neuron in the brain, we cannot read off the subjective experience, as the mapping between neural substrate and meaning is likely to be individualized. The only way to make further sense is by comparing the sets of neurons activated during subjectively meaningful circumstances *in the same individual a short while ago*: 'When I perceive the blue sky, this set of neurons is activated. Now the same set of neurons is activated when I am imagining, I infer that I am vividly imaging the colour of the blue sky'. In this scenario, it is necessary to invoke individualized subjective experience (blue sky perception) as a 'calibration' reference in the interpretation of brain data (the set of neurons activated). It is also necessary to specify the brief time frame to acknowledge the cumulative unfolding of both subjective experience and connections in the brain. Isolated empirical brain data on their own therefore cannot be expected to give total access to subjective experience.

Let us consider a further illustration with 'the act of winking', as proposed by the Oxford philosopher Gilbert Ryle (Geertz, 1973; Ryle, 1968). The wink of an eye can be viewed and described from different perspectives. Suppose you close your eyelids for a moment. First, we have to decide whether this is a voluntary act (a wink), a spontaneous act (a blink), or a reactive act (a blink reaction to a stimulus). How can we be sure it is a voluntary act? We have to ask the subject (i.e., you). However, your confirmation is not in the domain of Natural Science because you 'subjectively feel' that you have initiated the act. No other observer can penetrate your subjective experience and confirm 'objectively' that you have initiated the act. Indeed, it has been observed in pathological situations that we may *retrospectively* attribute an act to voluntary intentions (see section 8.4.3). Some may advocate using an 'intention' rating scale so that a number can represent your judgement of how 'intentional' the act was. As we see, this does not really add much information. We can measure the eye movements using electromyography and electrophysiology. It may be possible to tell the difference if we detect brain wave changes prior to the eye movement. If these brain wave changes are associated with voluntary initiation of eye movements *on other occasions* (e.g., possibly, the Readiness Potential, Kornhuber & Deecke, 1965; Libet, 1985), we can infer, using the *other occasions* as reference, that this is a voluntary blink. You, of course, will still have to reassure others that you did voluntarily initiate the wink on those *initial reference occasions*. This is only the beginning step in understanding the phenomenon of a wink. We then have to understand your subjective mental state in which you initiated the wink. Was it a signal to someone? What was the meaning of the signal? Did you wink to release some tension? Or to suppress an itch in the eye? To capture these phenomena, there is no alternative to the direct communication of your subjective experience.

1.1.5 Alternatives to positivist approaches

Mankind has also been seeking to understand the world and themselves through means other than empirical approaches. Such approaches contrast with the rationalist view that reason provides the only legitimate access to knowledge. Many thinkers believed that the rationalist approach may not provide us with full knowledge in the realm of human experience. Instead, the scientific study of the world via objective experimentation offers only one of the many possible ways of knowing (e.g., Searle, 1984).

1.1.6 Extreme responses to empirical limitations

In response to the limitations of the Natural Sciences in addressing subjective experience, Critchley (2001) pointed out that there are risks of falling into the extremes of either 'Naturalism' or 'Obscurantism'. 'Naturalism' believes that the scientific approach can be applied to understand 'everything that is worth understanding'. We have seen that such a view leads to an inadequate treatment of the less objectifiable human experiences.

'Obscurantism', on the other hand, proposes that human subjective phenomena cannot be reliably accessed. As a result, subjectivity is not open to reason and consistent knowledge cannot be pursued.

Both of these extremes can be avoided. We shall forward a notion that, with care, it is possible to handle subjective phenomena in a valid manner.

1.2 A Phenomenological Approach to Subjective Experiences

Phenomenology is the study of subjective experiences (phenomena) as they appear to a person. It could be one of the most direct ways of knowing as our own subjective experiences are immediately accessible to us.

Phenomenology is 'a descriptive science of whatever appears in subjective experience' (Husserl, 1913, 1921/1970). Phenomena are 'simply the ways things appear to an individual'. We note that phenomenology has a different foundation from the Natural Sciences. Phenomenology is founded on a careful observation and description of subjective experiences.

The discipline of phenomenology encompasses a broad range of activities (including Husserl's later positions). These initiatives are diverse and have developed different approaches to accommodate different applications. For our account, the framework of early Husserlian phenomenology is a pragmatic starting point. This approach treats subjective experiences as primary phenomena. Experience is mediated by mental representations situated between the individual and their world. We will also follow this framework as was articulated by Husserl's first assistant Edith Stein (later Saint Theresa Benedicta of the Cross) and consider her development of a phenomenology of empathy, in the context of a comprehensive account of the human person.

1.2.1 The Lifeworld and subjective experiences

The Lifeworld (*Lebenswelt*) (Husserl, 1936/1954) for a person is the world that is experienced directly by him subjectively in everyday life. The content of the Lifeworld is a result of the interaction between the individual and the 'external world', resulting in entities that are experienced subjectively. This Lifeworld is not exactly the same as the 'empirical' world. The structure of the empirical world can be accessed by Natural Sciences studies. In contrast, the Lifeworld consists of what is presented to the mind and is subjectively experienced. Husserl asserted that the Lifeworld can also be studied systematically. According to Husserl's (1936/1954) view, mankind engages in a wide range of experience in which scientific study is but one amongst many possible ways of knowing. While affirming the values of empirical science, it may also be helpful to consider whether a range of knowing is possible in understanding human experiences. In particular, we note that phenomenology aspires to systematically study human experiences as presented to their subjective mind.

1.2.2 The Lifeworld can be communicated through a dialogue

Psychopathology is concerned with subjective experiences that are disrupted by mental disorders. A phenomenological approach enables us to grasp the ways in which the Lifeworlds of individuals are shattered by mental illnesses (see section 2.5.2). Language is the *primary* medium through which these experiences can be communicated. We propose that it is through language that individual experience becomes partly sharable and thus *objectifiable* (see section 1.4.3). Psychopathological investigations involve skilled use of language to clarify anomalous subjective experiences (symptoms) in an informative and reliable manner (see section 1.3).

1.3 Some Cognitive Approaches to Subjective Phenomena

1.3.1 The importance of contextual meaning

Just as phenomenology has been trying to appreciate human experience from the 'inside', cognitive science has been trying to understand psychology from the 'outside'. We are particularly interested in where the two approaches converge.

   Switching to an observer's stance, Fodor (1978) regarded 'mental states' as the 'interplay between individuals and their mental representations'. Mental representations are constructed in the mind based on what actually is in the outside world (to represent it more, or less, accurately). The mind does not interact directly with the outside world but instead interacts through mental representations. Significantly, Fodor also recognized that mental representations can be articulated through linguistic expressions with sentence structures. Brain structure and brain function are considered to interact to give rise to consciousness (Fodor, 1968). Brain structure is considered as 'hardware' while brain function is considered as 'software'. Importantly, Fodor also proposed that there are different 'modules' in the mind. Each module handles a class of information relatively independently of other modules. These modules are defined according to their functions instead of their locations in the brain (Fodor, 1983).

   Searle (1980) considered this view further. His well-known Chinese post-room metaphor emphasized that having a processing algorithm (such as a computer software, as Fodor suggested above) is not sufficient for human understanding (Searle, 1980). He imagined a man who did not know the Chinese language but was taking his position in a post office where he had to sort letters according to addresses written in Chinese. He was instructed with a detailed set of rules that was able to cover all possible addresses. Although the man inside the Chinese post-room (with unlimited capacity for memory) could execute the expected sorting action based on an algorithm, he still cannot be said to 'know what the words mean' (semantics). *Meaning* can still be missing in such an algorithm-based process; that is, the man in the Chinese post room is not aware of the *meaning* of the Chinese words. Due to the absence of meaning, doubts are raised on whether algorithms and structures are sufficient to give rise to experience. It appears that access to meaning (see Chapter 5) is a necessary requirement for human experiences. The key advantage of a meaning system over an algorithm is related to the richness of mutually interacting connections, which provides flexible responses *even when the stimulus has not been encountered before* (see section 1.3.2). As we shall see, access to meaning is indeed critical for understanding experiences in health and in illness. Some psychopathological states are characterized by anomalous processing of meaning.

1.3.2 Cognitive theories of subjective experiences

Many cognitive accounts for conscious experience have been offered (e.g., Crick, 1994). We shall sample just a few and summarize some common features amongst them. A typical example is the Global Workspace Theory (Baars, 2002). It describes a 'fleeting memory capacity' that accesses different brain processes that are otherwise working in a parallel and distributed way (Baars, 1997). Similarly, the Conscious Awareness System (Schacter, 1989) proposes a brain module responsible for integrating information from a number of other cognitive modules, making them available to conscious awareness.

   The common theme these accounts share appears to be a central coordinating system with limited capacity, interacting with multiple information channels. The central coordinating system can link up with diverse cognitive modules and integrate information derived from them (see Searle's Chinese post room metaphor in section 1.3.1). We shall observe that these features may converge with the structure of subjective experience derived from phenomenological observations (see Chapter 3).

1.4 Summary: A Coherent Approach for Psychopathology?

1.4.1 The Lifeworld as a field of study

The question of whether the psychopathology of subjective experience can be positioned as a valid field of study requires careful consideration. We have seen that a simple assertion that subjective phenomena can be measured using empirical methodology borrowed from the Natural Sciences (such as rating scales) is inadequate. On the other hand, it also appears premature to assume that no objectifiable (shareable) knowledge can emerge from studies of subjective experience (see sections 1.1.1 and 1.1.2). This position would have discarded subjective experience as entirely beyond the reach of shared human knowledge.

A disciplined approach to psychopathology relies on a careful use of dialogue processes (see section 1.2.2). Through the anchoring of mutually aligned linguistic concepts, individuals can reliably and meaningfully communicate subjective experiences. Because of the shared semantic anchor, individual experiences map to a communal reality (Husserl, 1936/1954). Language therefore brings a kind of 'objectivity' to otherwise private experiences through the possibility of referencing within a shared semantic framework (see section 1.4.3). To the extent that subjective experience can be anchored by shared linguistic markers (i.e., words), they are open to investigation and can be explored in an *objective* manner; that is, they are more than completely private experiences. The referencing to a shared semantic frame in which the linguistic categories are located becomes an important foundation for descriptive psychopathology (Jaspers, 1913/1963). Alongside psychopathology, a related discipline has been developed in anthropology. Ethnography has elaborated on the concept of 'thick description' in which the observer 'immerses' himself intensely in an unfamiliar environment in order to access the meaning reference in which linguistic categories and experiences were expressed (Geertz, 1973). In psychopathology the process of the 'verstehen' has a similar goal (Jasper, 1913/1963). The interviewer employs his capacity for empathic understanding and uses the meaning inherent in his immersion experience to provide reference for the semantic contents expressed by the subject (see Chapter 5). It is important to recognize that these processes are made possible through the mediation of language.

1.4.2 The grasp of subjective experience in psychopathology

In summary, subjective experiences are not fully accessible 'from the outside' using empirical techniques from the brain sciences. Also, adequate access is not fully attained through the empirical social science techniques such as questionnaires (see section 1.1.1). These methods need to be accompanied by a more engaging approach to gain appropriate access to subjective experience.

It is proposed here that meaningful access to subjective data is possible through a disciplined use of the dialogue process (the Clinical Dialogue, see Chapter 9). Mediation of language is crucial in this process. Through disciplined use of dialogues as tools, meaningful and reliable information can emerge. It is possible to extract reliable information from the experiential data provided by the subjects through a shared linguistic frame (see section 1.4.3).

1.4.3 Language mediates access to psychopathology

Semantic concepts provide a map of the Lifeworld (including the self, others, and the physical world), which can be shared between individuals (see section 1.4.1) (Nowak

& Krakauer, 1999; Solé et al., 2010). The relationship between concepts is often ordinal rather than metric in nature (e.g., hot>warm>cold, rather than degrees Celsius). Language can chart ordinal relationships on the semantic map. Such anchoring relationships can be confirmed in qualitative agreements between individuals.

Besides expressing relations and comparisons, some words have a direct mapping to verifiable objects in the external world (explicit referents, e.g., the sun). These words are shared between individuals. Some words are not directly linked to shared observations but are weaved in with the explicit referent words through ordinal anchoring relationships. As a result, experiences can be mapped consistently between individuals who share these words. Thus, through the mediation of language, subjective experiences become (partially) communicable.

We have laboured on the accessibility of subjective experience to vigorous empirical knowing and have suggested that it is possible through clarification via language processes. This point is not just to support the obvious importance of empathic understanding in therapeutic interactions. Quite separately, we are suggesting that skilful access to subjective experience may provide reliable information to enhance the understanding and treatment of mental disorders.

This position is not trivial and may in fact almost be surprising in a 'materialistic' era where digital outputs are generally more valued than human communications. Let us consider the following example. In enhancing more accurate detection of mental illnesses before their full-blown manifestation (i.e., in the at-risk mental state), much attention and resources have been invested on the use of 'digital phenotypes' and 'machine learning' to help uncover potential but hidden biological information. At the same time, scanty attention has been paid to accurately clarify the phenomena that the subjects are experiencing. We advocate paying more attention to the subjective phenomena. Currently, the rating scales typically used in such studies are relatively crude. It will be empirically enlightening to see to what extent prediction accuracy can be improved by more detailed phenomenological analysis.

1.4.4 Conclusion

In this chapter, we first highlighted the fact that psychopathology involves human subjective experience. We raised the awareness that the study of subjective experience may be different from the study of Natural Science objects. We then proposed that a simple adoption of the empirical method is inadequate for psychopathology. We next reviewed possible strategies in anchoring a 'human' domain of knowledge. In this context we also rejected the paralysing position that reliable information cannot be obtained at all in the subjective phenomena. We suggested that human experience can be reliably communicated through a disciplined use of language. Exploration of subjective experience is possible through a skilled dialogue process. With this insight, we reappraised phenomenology as a reliable approach to study anomalous human subjective experience. In the coming chapters, we shall explore the convergent interaction between phenomenology and other disciplines in understanding the human mind. While we concluded that human subjective experience cannot be fully understood by describing empirical brain processes alone, we also rejected an approach that disregards brain processes as being irrelevant in understanding human experience. We shall proceed to build up an account of subjective experience that is informed (but not exhausted) by empirical knowledge of the brain. Our first step is to ask what aspect of knowledge about the brain is most likely to be relevant to the understanding of subjective experience.

2

Information in the Brain and Subjective Experiences

2.1 Overview

In this chapter, starting with an assumption that at least some aspects of subjective experience are related to brain states, we embark upon a broad reflection over the biological functions of the human brain. Numerous attempts have been made to map externally measured brain states to experiences, with limited successes. In this section, we are not going into details of these endeavours. Instead, we are going to start with a broad perspective addressing the functions of the human brain, appreciating the brain as one of the organs in the human body. In this way, our modest starting perspective is a reappraisal of the ordinary functions of the brain as an organ.

Without some ideas of what functions the human brain is meant to be serving, it is difficult to understand how the processes involved may go wrong. We begin by considering the role of the brain in 'handling information'. This perspective leads us to examine more broadly the nature of 'information transfer' in biological systems and cognitive systems. We note the difference between 'informational' and 'material' objects. Tools for studying 'information' are not yet as well developed as those available for studying material objects. These broader considerations reveal that information transfer is fundamental not only to the human mind but also to other organ systems and indeed to living organisms in general. We arrive at an appreciation that biological systems are characterized as much by 'information transfer' as by material exchanges. Information becomes increasingly important along evolutionary developments of life forms that eventually led to the emergence of the human mind. We also consider the artificial environment generated by human inventions being partly material but also partly informational. Rapid advances in human technology are producing a vastly expanded informational world in which human experiences can dwell.

We propose that subjective experiences correspond to information received in the mind via 'mental representations' (see Fodor's representational theory of mind in section 1.3.1). Mental representations are structures that hold organized information as coherent experiential contents. Inherent in the idea of 'holding' is the recognition that the same structure (form) can potentially be filled with different contents at different times. We consider 'information generation' as the process of selecting specific contents for filling the 'representation structures'. We propose a simple model (in the form of parallel distributed systems) as a pragmatic tool for modelling mental representations and their information transfer processes (Rumelhart et al., 1987). Such systems are based upon multiple interconnected processing units organized in a structure broadly consistent with the organization of neural units in the brain (parallel processing using distributed representations, see section 2.3.1). Even though they are not intended for detailed modelling of physiological brain processes, their emergent behaviours exhibit features that provide converging accounts consistent with phenomenological observations of subjective experiences.

These considerations of the functions of the brain lead us to an appreciation of the rapidly changing artificial environment (in an evolution time scale) that humans have created, yet the human brain may find itself struggling to catch up. This situation raises issues with an understanding of brain dysfunction in terms of biological utility in adaptation to a changing environment. In generating a more embracing framework, the ideas of 'relating' and 'health' emerged. This exploration starts with examining the functions of the brain. It ends with concluding remarks concerning some higher features dimensions in human experience (such as 'well-being') relevant to psychopathology.

2.2 What Does Information Mean in Physical, Biological, and Semantic Systems?

The brain handles information, not material. Material occupies space and time and is conserved (i.e., material cannot be created from nothing or vanish and cannot be indefinitely multiplied). Information does not occupy space or time and can be multiplied without apparent limit. The brain is unique amongst organs in the human body in its specialization to handle information rather than material. In the brain, energy is consumed to sustain systems (such as neuronal networks) that manage information. Information is expressed in the brain as the selective activation of neural units and the modification of connections between them (Morris, 1989), leading to changes in behavioural choice or experiences. The human brain is adapted for interacting with information in specific ways and can be considered as an 'information-consuming' organ (Pylyshyn, 1984). Information in the brain is considered as the basis for subjective experience in the mind.

2.2.1 Information in physical systems

To understand the roles played by the brain in handling information, we shall start with a more detailed examination of the question, 'what is information?'. This question is not trivial and has inspired several treaties (e.g., Gleick, 2011). We shall keep to a simple pragmatic account relevant to understanding the role of information in psychopathology.

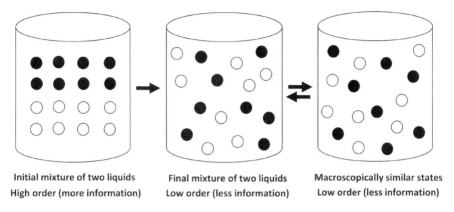

Initial mixture of two liquids   Final mixture of two liquids   Macroscopically similar states
High order (more information)   Low order (less information)   Low order (less information)

Figure 2.1. The concept of 'information' illustrated by the mixing of two liquids (e.g., milk and tea, with their molecules represented, respectively, by black and white dots). From left to right the diagrams represent (1) the initial mixture when the two liquids are largely separate (the information state is high, it is difficult to randomly arrive at this state) and (2) the final mixture when after a period of spontaneous settling the two liquids are well-mixed (black and white dots are well-mixed, the information state is low as it is likely that random movements of black and white dots will arrive in one of the many equivalent states, i.e., the black and white dots in different, random positions, but from the outside the mixed liquid is no different). The two-way arrows between the middle and the right diagrams show the changes between different 'equivalent states' (black and white dots in different positions but still well-mixed). The information in these states is low as it is easy for the system to randomly arrive at one of the many similar 'equivalent states', which look exactly the same externally. With time, most isolated physical systems tend to settle in such low information states because of random molecular movements (see section 2.2.1).

In a broad sense, information may be considered as a measure of 'order' (level of organization or complexity) in a system (Shannon, 1948). The opposite of information is 'disorder' in a system (Brooks et al., 1988). A system that is less specified (i.e., where multiple possibilities are open) is considered to be more disorderly and 'low' in information (Feynman et al., 1963; Prigogine, 1967). In communication (a specific case of information transfer), the information state in the recipient system changes upon arrival of signals from the sender system. The signals result in the recipient system becoming more specified (i.e., more disposed towards a specific response).

We further illustrate what is meant by a system 'being more specified'. A simple example is a mixture of two liquids (e.g., black tea and milk) settling over a period of time (see Figure 2.1). After settling, the mixture, milk tea, becomes stable from moment to moment, as there is no change in its *macroscopic* form. Even though the exact molecular particles (microscopic states) change constantly (e.g., in Figure 2.1(a), whether a particle in a particular location is black or white), they do not alter the macroscopic properties of the mixture (the populations of black and white particles, though in different positions, are still uniformly distributed). In this sense, the different microscopic molecular states are equivalent to one another macroscopically. The large number of equivalent states corresponding to a well-mixed liquid (e.g., the milk tea) means that the system is likely to align by chance with one instance of this large set of possible states. Because of the large number of possible equivalent states, this macroscopic set of states is regarded as being a lower informational state (see Figure 2.1(b) and 2.1(c)). In other words, it is easier to end up in one of these states by chance. In contrast, if the two liquids are well segregated, as in the initial juxtaposition before mixing (e.g., when the milk has just been added to the tea, not yet mixed), only a small number of possible microscopic configurations correspond to these states (see Figure 2.1(a)). They are highly unlikely to be arrived at by chance. These states, being less likely to emerge as a random outcome, are considered as carrying a larger amount of information (see Figure 2.1). In this way, the measure of order can be described: in a physical system, with the random movement in molecules, there is a gradual loss of information with the passage of time (see Figure 2.2).

We can make use of this example to explore the relationship between non-random (correlated) phenomena and information. Suppose the movements of molecules are not entirely random, in that a certain molecule tends to move together with certain other molecules. There is then a correlation within the observed phenomena. The correlation results in a reduction in the number of possible states. The observation of correlations or associations is therefore associated with an increase in information and a reduction of the number of possible states in a system. More generally, information can be considered as conditional probability: if A is present, then the number of possible states in B is reduced (i.e., the information is increased, randomness is reduced).

In physical systems, order generally decreases with time because of random molecular movements. In contrast, in biological systems, information often increases with more order being accrued with time (Adami et al., 2000; Brooks et al., 1988). Information also appears to increase with time in cognitive/semantic systems (see section 2.2.3).

2.2.2 Information in biological systems

How is information embedded in biological systems? Physiological processes in the body are usually measured in terms of quantitative variables in physics and chemistry (e.g., mole, grams, metres). The heart pumps a volume of blood into the arteries. The liver enables chemical reactions along metabolic pathways. The kidneys regulate electrolyte and urea concentrations. These systems involve material substances, and the Natural Sciences have developed the corresponding quantitative measurements. In contrast, the brain deals with information, which does not occupy space and has no mass. The basic sciences for studying information (i.e., cybernetics and computational science) are not yet as familiar as physics and chemistry.

In the brain, information is stored as neural connections that specify propensities for behavioural responses (Baddeley et al., 1999). Behaviourally, information is expressed as the narrowing down of response possibilities in a given situation. Experientially, information increase is associated with the subjective awareness of transitions from the unknown to the known, from the uncertain to the certain, and from the unpredictable to the more predictable. Experiential increase in information is a process that unfolds continuously throughout an individual's life.

In fact, we can revisit other physiological processes in the human body and observe that they actually share the same general tendency towards producing an increase in orderliness and a reduction of randomness (Stark & Theodoridis, 1973). Be it in the filtering action of the kidneys, in the chemical reactions in the liver, the pumping actions of the blood, or the wiring of the brain, order is ultimately increased in the maintenance of a constant internal milieu against changing external conditions (i.e., the phenomena referred to as homeostasis, Bernard, 1865/1974). Order is embedded in the gradients of chemical concentrations, in molecular bonds, and in cellular processes (e.g., in the immune system). These processes stop with the cessation of life. After life departs, the body of an organism follows physical laws in the process of disintegration. In life, the brain plays the same role of increasing organization complexity just as other organs in the body. It is unique in that it organizes ideas and behavioural likelihood rather than tangible material substances. The main difference is that the brain is developed with highly adaptive units (neuronal networks) in which the material constraints are minimized in exchange for representational capability. They are therefore adapted to representing complex and diverse items in the external world (from material objects to ideas). In constructing mental representations, the actual material basis is not decisive; that is, the mental representations can be based on alternative material systems other than neurons and synapses and serve the same contents.

2.2.3 Information in semantic systems: From material to information

In the last section, we observed that, in contrast to physical systems, in living systems, information and order increase with time. In this section, we consolidate this notion by contrasting in more detail information handling in three systems: physical systems, biological systems, and human experience (or semantic systems) (see Figure 2.2). We shall also consider the interactions between these systems. This comparison provides a context for considering information generation as a key process in subjective human life.

In physical systems, the trend for a gradual reduction of order is based on random movement in molecular units (see section 2.2.1). Biological organisms are built from physical components and share the inevitable trend towards physical disorder. However, biological systems also contain two mechanisms for counteracting the tendencies towards disorder. The first is physiological homeostatic mechanisms, which keep the body in an organized internal milieu. The second is self-replicating mechanisms (see

Figure 2.2). The theory of evolution proposed that random generation of biological diversity through mutation could subsequently be selected by nature, with the selected features being perpetuated by self-replication.

Semantic systems (cognitive systems with 'meaning') concern information conveyed as ideas and concepts. A basic unit of information in the mind is the observation of correlations (associations) amongst objects and ideas. The brain can be viewed as a platform for dealing with complex associations (Wernicke, 1881/2005). Correlation can be expressed in the following form: given feature A, the probability of feature B is increased. The human mind explores and discovers correlation patterns in the world. This same activity becomes highly specialized in empirical scientific observations. It leads to increasingly complex knowledge about the world.

The platform where the biological semantic systems play out is the brain. Ideas also contain their own self-replication mechanisms (see Figure 2.2). New ideas are generated and selected. Ideas (as organized information) can be conserved by selective retention and dissemination (e.g., Blackmore, 1999). This can take place in the brain and increasingly also on paper and in the digital medium.

In physical systems, high-information (order) systems gradually lose order (and information) as they inevitably become increasingly random. In biological systems, there is an increase in information (and order) with individual life (homeostasis) and with natural selection of species. Adaptation to the environment drives the direction for the increase in order. When individual life expires, the body follows the rules of a physical system and 'returns to dust'. In semantic systems, symbols and ideas are selected in individual semantic systems in the mind (which is supported by the biological system). Cultural interaction between individuals determines the propagation of ideas in a population. Ideas may eventually result in changes in the environment, thus influencing the direction of development in the biological system.

We observe that in both the biological system and the semantic system 'entities' can be preserved and developed over time. The capacity for replication of forms and the interaction with a selecting environment are conditions that counteract the progression towards a random state of disorder. In such 'order-generating' systems, a selecting environment coupled with a replication mechanism can generate new orderliness over time.

In this way, the environment imposes 'information' that shapes the growth direction of a system through selection (Davies, 1999). With time, the adapted outcomes of earlier selection themselves become new features embedded in the environment to determine the future selection of new 'forms' in subsequent organisms (see Figure 2.2). For example, in the tropical forest, the competition for light for photosynthesis in a crowded biomass encourages the development of dense foliage on trees. The dense foliage themselves subsequently become the shaping environments (light is depleted in the space beneath them) that encourage the success of trees with more elevated foliage. Their success changes the environment to favour elevated foliage. This new environment in turn shapes the development of animals that can reach the elevated foliage

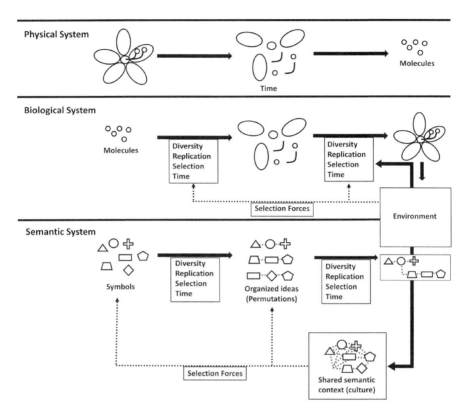

Figure 2.2. Information exchanges in physical, biological, and semantic systems and their interactions. With time, high information (complexity) physical systems gradually lose complexity (and information) as they inevitably become increasingly random. In biological systems, there is an increase in information (and order) in the individual lifetime (growth and homeostasis), as well as with natural selection of biological species over the evolution time scale. New features (information) adaptive to the environment can appear through natural selection with an increase in information. When individual life expires, the body follows the rules of a physical system and 'returns to dust'. In semantic systems, ideas are selected in an individual's brain (which is supported by the biological system). Cultural interaction between individuals determines the propagation of ideas in a population. Ideas may eventually result in changes in the environment (e.g., the development of technology). This can affect the environment and influence the direction of evolution in the biological system (see section 2.2).

for food (e.g., the giraffe). The same principles apply to the evolution of ideas in an individual and the evolution of culture in a population of individuals. Ideas survive in the individual based on how they interact with other ideas in the same individual. Ideas survive in a community (culture) based on how well they fit in with existing ideas in the population. We note that the human brain is the physical milieu in which selection of ideas takes place. The human brain is itself a product of evolution for *Homo sapiens* in a prehistoric environment. Cultural ideas, although themselves not tangible, have led to actions of sapiens with concrete impacts on the environment. They have brought about agriculture, domestication of animals, urbanization, reading, text, industrial revolution, and digital technology. We shall see that for human beings, the rapid development of culture has accelerated the changes in the human living environment at a rate that arguably may have outpaced the biological evolution of the human brain.

Physical, biological, and semantic systems interact. Physical systems exhibit an inevitable trend towards randomness. Biological systems are composed of physical materials. The molecules that make up biological individuals are also subjected to the same trends. As a result, the individual organisms move towards disintegration and eventually 'return to dust' (see Figure 2.2). However, despite the demise of individuals, the species 'lives on'. What is a species? The species is not just a collection of individuals. A species is not specified by individuals; it is a 'form' shared by individuals, including those not yet born. This 'form' is what is preserved in biology. The 'form' lies in the realm of 'information', not materials. This emphasis on information is important in our further consideration of psychopathology in subjective experiences.

Biology studies living forms. Biological forms are informational and not material. Although 'forms' are expressed in transient individual existence, they are independent of individual material existence. It is deceptively easy to overlook this and misconceive biology as dealing with living substances because the life span of many commonly encountered biological organisms are comparable to our own. It is only when we contemplate a larger timescale that we appreciate the transience of the individuals in relation to the persistence of their biological forms (species). This exploration also enables us to appreciate the value that lies in the 'informational' rather than the 'material' aspects of life. In a 'materialistic' age, it is refreshing to revisit this issue and recognize that much of what is interesting and important in life lies in the 'information' rather than the 'material' realm.

Having harnessed ourselves with an appreciation of the informational realm as being fundamental to what is salient in human life, we return to the notion that the information in the brains of individuals underlies individual subjective experiences. Human experience is assumed to be dependent on the biology of the brain and does not exist apart from the brain (which is a biological 'form') (Andrieu, 2006). However, some aspects of human experience can be shared with others so that the information can persist independently of individual brains (Andrieu, 2006). We consider such a sharable aspect of human experience as belonging to 'culture'. Culture in turn becomes the context for shaping individual experiences (see Figure 2.2).

2.2.3.1 *Information handling exchange between the individual brain and collective culture*

How does information flow through an individual's brain? Can new information be created? What governs the transfer of information between the individual and his environment?

In the individual, life experience and knowledge accumulate during development and education, and this results in an increase in information for the individual (Dretske, 1981). Some of these can be communicated to others, and thereby contribute to cultural contents. The gradual accumulation of cultural information involves a two-way interaction between the individual mind and the collective culture. In the individual brain, information accumulated over a lifetime contributes to the increase in specification of mental contents for an individual until the mind is no longer capable of storing new information due to aging processes. Some information in the individual mind can be imparted to other minds. This shared information (culture) can last beyond the life of the individual.

Creative processes involve the net production of new information. Novel ideas are positioned amongst existing ideas. The relationship between the novel ideas and existing ideas acts as a selection filter to determine the survival of the new ideas. New ideas that are coherent with old ideas are retained and further developed (see the account on memes by Blackmore, 1999; Dawkins, 1976). Ideas that do not fit well are discarded. Creative processes are involved in the production of mutually supporting clusters of new ideas. When a coherent assembly of budding ideas emerges, there is a further quantum increase in information (i.e., a paradigm shift, Kuhn, 1962). These processes are not necessarily fulfilled in all individuals. There is a cessation of information gain when one fails to acquire new information in life. There is also a lack of contribution of information to culture when an individual withdraws from society.

Cultural communication can be mediated by words or by actions (e.g., behaving in a certain manner). Owing to the possibility of easy deception with words, action has been viewed as being more 'authentic', albeit with less efficiency of dissemination. This situation may change with progress in digital communication technology. The advent of online videos allows compelling images of 'actions' to be widely and quickly disseminated.

The generation of information by individuals, as well as the flow of information between individuals and the group, constitutes the fundamental functions of the brain. Ill health can critically compromise these processes.

2.2.4 The brain as an organ for holding complex contextual information

We shall review the concepts of 'information' so far discussed. Having unpacked the concept of 'information', we shall consider how the concept of 'context' is relevant to understanding how 'information' is handled in the brain. The notion of 'information' has been used in two ways:

(1) The first perspective for 'information' is as a measure of the level of organization in a system. In this sense, 'information' contained in a particular 'state' in a system is related to how likely this particular state can be 'arrived at' through a random process. A system that is 'less-specified', that is, more likely to be arrived at by random processes (because it has more equivalent molecular states, like in a homogenous mixture), is considered to be less organized and contains less information. A system that is highly unique, and corresponds to a high degree of specification (i.e., has few equivalent micro/molecular states, so that it is less likely to be arrived at by random movement of molecules), contains more information. The amount of information change is specifiable as the difference in the number of possible equivalent states. In this sense, information is defined as the number of possible states. Related to this sense of information is the phenomenon of correlation between features. In a more organized system, there are correlations between different elements. The specified condition in one feature constrains the probable condition in another feature. This makes the system more predictable. A system specified by internal correlations contains more information. In the process of learning, the individual discovers correlated patterns in the environment. Successful learning will result in a more informative model of the environment, allowing more accurate prediction to take place.

(2) The second construct of 'information' is as signals conveyed in a 'communication' process. In this sense, 'information' is about messages that are 'sent' by an agent and 'received' by another agent. Here, information refers to the extent to which the signal content received by the recipient is conveyed as it is 'intended' by the sender.

Importantly, in this view, 'information' as 'what is being communicated' involves a 'sender' and a 'recipient'. Although in the classical sense, the senders and recipients are assumed to be persons, this need not be the case. Senders and recipients in an information system can be biological, digital, or mechanical. Regardless, recipients are required to have 'sensors' that are designed to detect signals. Whether the recipients have received the relevant signals usually needs to be inferred from the behaviour of the recipient. Behaviours in response to signals are observed in line with the following conditions:

(a) There exist a number of different potential behaviour options, out of which one is eventually selected, for example, a movement possibility in several different directions.

(b) The choice is not random but dependent to varying extents on external and internal environments; these factors modify the probability of the selection of a particular option (e.g., more likely to be moving towards one of the possible directions).

(c) Signals can be detected by sensors in the agent.

To show that information transfer has taken place, some changes in the response choice need to be observed as a result of the arrival of the signal. This system does not presuppose conscious awareness and can be applied to lower animals, plants, and non-biological systems.

In random responses (e.g., in Brownian movements), no information is involved (probabilities of different movement directions are equal; i.e., the direction of movement is random). 'Information' is evidenced by selective responsiveness to the environment (e.g., to light or food). This involves the selection of a particular movement direction in the presence of a stimulus (e.g., light or food). In this situation, the response options are selective (i.e., the probability are not evenly distributed), though not necessarily totally deterministic (these systems can still be probabilistic). In this framework, the above two notions of 'information', that of order in a system and that of communication content, are related coherently.

'Information' that influences response in a system can either be 'simple' stimulus (a foreground signal) or it can be a 'complex' background information that is considered 'contextual' (or conditional on a number of mutually related factors). Contexts do not directly provoke responses; instead, they modify the responses to other stimuli.

Nervous systems in higher organisms act as a 'holder of multiple possible contexts'. Context influences the conditional possibilities in the selection of a behaviour in response to incoming stimuli. Contextual information results in 'reduction in possibilities'.

Momentary incoming sensory information interacts with background contextual information to determine a behavioural response. Foreground sensory input is put side by side with background input from the external environment (external context), as well as with information in memory (internal context) (Goldstein, 1939).

The different components in the external world are not totally independent of one another. There are inbuilt patterns in the external, empirical natural world. The basic relationship between these patterns is observed as an association (correlation) between two features. That some features of the environment are specifically correlated with others, with uneven probability (i.e., more than by chance), reflects the underlying structure in nature. Such associative structure is informative (i.e., contains information) as it specifies a subset of 'actual world' feature configurations amongst all possible configurations. Constraints in the real world reduce possible permutations. After one feature emerges (e.g., footprints of a bear), the probability that a particular next feature (a bear) will follow is not random. This forms the basis of empirical knowledge about the external world.

Complex contextual information can be built up from cascades of multiple components. It is held in memory as semantic contents. The integration of multiple contextual information may lead to simplification (e.g., in categorization) and to the discovery of generalizable associations (e.g., laws of nature). These associations help to capture predictable patterns in the world.

The human mind encodes and holds a complex contextual environment through mental constructs assembled using the generative capacity of language and the tenacity of concepts. When we are conscious of these constructs, we call them 'ideas'. There may be aggregates of associated features that act as context but are not explicitly articulable in terms of linguistic concepts or ideas. They nevertheless produce an effect on the behaviour choice of the individual. We call these 'representational fragments'. 'Meaning' refers to the coherent activation of a network of related representations including associated emotional and action features.

The mind's capacity of handling sequential linguistic representations (in which units are arranged in a linear order) is limited. Massively parallel representations and limited-capacity sequential handling of linguistic categories compete for resource allocation in the brain. The ability to reduce the number of feature dimensions in constructs becomes important. Some of the more complex information is reduced to simpler ideas that can be more readily handled by the mind using a structure supported by human linguistic capacities.

The usefulness of a mental construct lies in how well it explains and predicts the empirical world. Often multiple components are included in a prediction model. When a simple model nevertheless predicts the external world well, it is considered to be a more efficient representation of information (Occam's razor). Complex constructs are often involved when it is not feasible to predict empirical patterns more simply. They can be seen as attempts to fit existing data before more parsimonious underlying principles are 'discovered'. While they accommodate past data, they may not perform well in predicting the future.

Can information ever be created *de novo*? When a mind selects a direction in the way it handles content, or selects a response to a given stimulus in the environment, information is increased. Where does the new information come from? Was it 'created' *de novo*? Was the information already latent in what has been accumulated as stored contextual information in the mind? In other words, is it latent *in potentia* in the existing ideas and the relationship between these ideas? At a deeper level, solving a problem may not necessarily involve the *de novo* creation of new information. What is involved is a selected accumulation of ideas within an individual mind. The exact context that determines how ideas are selectively aggregated in an individual mind involves the interplay of a myriad of historical, social, and psychological factors.

The human brain has the unique capacity to hold together a large set of organized information, as 'potential contexts' that eventually may have impacts on behavioural output. Contextual information has also grown to be much richer and far more complex, with cascades of conditional relationships as the brain increases in capacity. The mind therefore is a platform for the re-combination, sorting, and refinement of ideas. In this process, salience, knowledge, categorization, and cultural identity each plays out their roles to distil and refine relevant ideas. The brain is capable of holding *in potentia* a large number of future possibilities. This includes potential configuration of ideas and contexts.

The brain allows past information and future possibilities to be held together for the selection of action in the present moment. Only the action in the present moment can have an impact on the world. Action involves selection and can be physical material, as well as communicative-informational. Action narrows down possibilities. The larger universe of collective human activities thus increases in information over time in a process of individual and collective evolution (i.e., history).

2.3 Mental Representations Are Containers of Information

Following the discourse on information flow in human life, we consider the proposal that information is handled in the brain/mind with 'mental representations' (Dretske, 1981; Markman & Dietrich, 2000).

Mental representations (mental models, concepts, or ideas) are bridges between the mind and objects in the external world. Ideas and concepts help the human mind handle objects by placing them within a coherent system of meaning. Representations (we use the terms 'representation' and 'mental representation' in an interchangeable way in this work) play a vital role in how we experience the world (Kempson, 1988). Mental representations can be simple, mapping directly to an external object, or complex, referring to states of affairs (SOAs) in the external world. Complex representations often have a propositional (language-like) structure.

One essential feature of the mind is its ability to represent. To represent means 'to stand in for one thing with another'. The mind can refer to, handle, and store

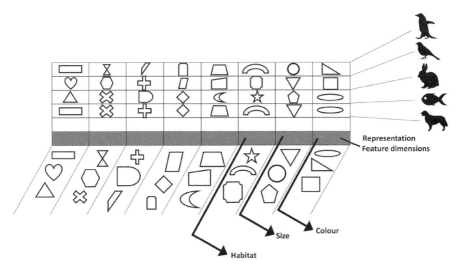

Figure 2.3. Mental representations as organized holders of information in the mind. The structure of a mental representation depicting groups of objects (i.e., categories, e.g., animals) can be visualized as a table with rows and columns. Columns represent features dimensions (e.g., habitat, size, and colour). Rows represent individual members within the category (e.g., rabbit, penguins, dogs). On a specific occasion, the dimensions can be 'filled' with specific contents (represented by the different shapes e.g., living in jungles, large, brown) to represent a specific member (see section 2.3).

'representations' of external and internal objects. The nature of mental representations has been explored from different perspectives. Most would agree that the brain (or cell assemblies in the brain) ultimately implements mental representations through activation patterns in neuronal populations. However, the assumption that representations 'supervene' on the brain does not necessarily reduce them to 'mere' brain processes. Some of the most useful models advanced to understand mental representations address them as computational structures (Dietrich, 2007). Computational models depict mental representations as data structures that are implemented by the brain's hardware (cell assemblies) and used by cognitive systems to handle objects in the environment. The information in the data is the representational content.

The brain appears to adopt a diverse range of mental representations. Mental representations can be grouped according to their functions, the domains in which the object they represent are located, the computational structure, or the operational mode. In terms of function, they can be related to perceptions, actions, or thinking (i.e., semantic actions) (see section 6.1). In terms of domain, representations may refer to objects in the 'empirically external' world, the world of ideas, the inner body, or the self. In terms of structure, representations can be characterized by whether they are simple or complex, conceptual or non-conceptual, discrete or analogous, language-like or image-like, symbolic or sub-symbolic, classical or connectionist, and so forth.

Mental representations are also dynamic structures. They can operate in a mode that is more influenced by other mental representations (mind-mind relation, internal reference) or in a mode more mapped onto objects in the external world (world-mind relations, external reference).

At any moment in time, mental representations can also be 'filled' or 'unfilled'. An unfilled representation is a template structure with a number of feature dimensions, set up in the cognitive space of the mind for handling incoming information. In the unfilled state it may represent a class of similar objects (e.g., small animals), the details of which may be specified further or left unfilled. A filled representation is one in which each of the feature dimensions has been specified by a specific instance (e.g., a rabbit in addition to being a small animal). An unfilled representation can interact with the environment and receive information in two distinct ways. Firstly, an object in the environment can fill a representation on a moment-by-moment basis. Secondly, after repeated exposures to similar objects, the representation can learn the pattern of activation; for example, feature A is more likely to be associated with feature B. This results in long-term acquisition of information from the environment, which is stored as connection weights within the pattern (see section 2.3.1). Filled representations denoting exemplars relate to unfilled representations denoting categories in a hierarchical manner. In the representations for categories, fewer feature dimensions are specified and a larger number of feature dimensions are free. In the representations for individual exemplar, more feature dimensions are fixed.

Low-level, image-like, representations are often directly linked to sensory input from the environment (Kosslyn, 1980). They are continuous analogue variables.

Low-level representations provide the basic components to build high-level, composite, language-like representations that are used in planning, learning, and problem solving. High-level representations often are organized in a propositional structure and use the semantic unit (concept) as discrete signals. Representations carry information about the environment (external), and different representations cross-reference each other in the semantic system (internal). Thinkers differ in their views on the relative importance of external and internal contributions. Mental representations supervene on (or are implemented by) brains just like word processors supervene on the computer hardware. However, mental representations may not be entirely reduced to brain processes, because some key features of mental representations may not be captured at the brain implementing level. (Dietrich used an excellent example of the spell-checker being implemented by the computer, but the phenomena of misspelling and the correction are not found in the level of hardware of the computer.) Similarly, mental representations may operate at their own levels with properties that are not accessed at the neural implementation levels (Dietrich, 2007).

Many models of mental representations have been proposed. These include Johnson-Laird's 'mental models' (1983), Minsky's 'frames' (1974), Kosslyn's 'quasi-pictures' (1980), and Smolensky's 'sub-symbolic structure' (1995). Amongst the different models, the two main camps are the classic model (Fodor, 1983; Marr, 1982; Newell & Simon, 1976; Pylyshyn, 1984; Turing, 1950) and the connectionist model (Rumelhart et al., 1987; Smolensky, 1988). In the classic representation model, basic units are enduring and discrete, and the operations are rule-based algorithms. In contrast, in the connectionist models, units are transient, distributed, and massively parallel. It is now clear that both classical and connectionist models are involved in mental representations at different levels. We shall adopt these main directions in our approach to mental representations.

A 'basic' representation is a structure corresponding to a single semantic unit, that is, a concept, referring to an object. It consists of a specified number of dimensions. Each dimension can be filled with a choice from a number of possible alternatives. A specific combination of chosen options in these feature dimensions characterizes the representation. For example, in the representation for 'birds', when the dimensions are specified as 'do not fly', 'large size', 'cold environment', 'black and white colour', this permutation of features characterizes a penguin-like bird (Rumelhart et al., 1987) (see Figure 2.3).

Mental representations can thus be considered as templates in the mind. Some representations are learnt and some are hardwired in the brain (Hurford, 2003). Representational structures can be repeatedly recycled, with the specific slots being filled on each occasion by different contents to represent different things and situations.

Information is specified by the determination of specific details that fill the slots in the representational templates (see Figure 2.3). Representations are important for understanding psychopathology, as they mediate between the mind and the 'external reality'. Often it is important to ask whether a pathological experience is mediated

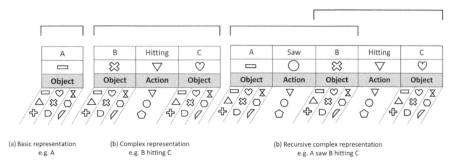

Figure 2.4. Basic and complex mental representations. Left: basic representation; middle: complex representation; right: recursive complex representation. Simple representation refers to a distinctive object. Complex representation represents a 'state of affairs' consisting of several objects and defining the relationship between them, often involving an 'action' in the relationship. Complex representations often have a language-like structure with a verb representing the relationship between the objects. Recursive complex representations are complex representation units with embedded representations. This is made possible by the language-like (propositional) structures of complex and recursive complex mental representations.

by changes in the structure of the representation itself (e.g., the number of features included) or whether it only affects the contents that are filling the representations.

To summarize our discussions so far, 'mental representations' are internal data structures in the mind that reflect some aspects of the world when filled with specific values. (In this work we use mental representation for both the unfilled template and the filled specific object; when usage is unclear, we shall add 'filled' or 'unfilled' to specify the meaning.) Representations are 'internal mental states analogous to data structures in computers, implemented in a brain's neural hardware, used by cognitive systems to navigate in, think about, and manipulate objects and processes found in their environment' (Dietrich, 2007). Mental representations act as intermediaries between the person's mind and the external world (Fodor, 1983). There are 'basic' representations for simple objects in the external world, as well as 'complex' representations for 'states of affairs' (SOAs) consisting of organized combinations of basic representations relating to one another (see Figure 2.4). Basic representations are often rich in perceptual features. Complex representations often have propositional structures that accommodate a number of constituent basic representations. Representations can also be not filled with perceptual details but are handled like conceptual units. It is possible that the quantity of perceptual details is constrained by limited capacity channels that handle propositional data structures.

Importantly, mental representations may contain more information than what is directly presented to the senses (Plotkin & Nowak, 2000). Apart from mediating experience, mental representations allow sapiens to represent 'things' that they have not directly experienced, and even 'things' that do not exist in the external world (Thompson & Byrne, 2002). Mental representations have been studied in detail in several areas (e.g., visual experiences) (Marr, 1982).

Information can be appreciated by inspecting processes that lead to information change. Information generation can be considered as a process of selecting more specific options out of a larger set of possibilities. Out of the many initial possibilities, a smaller number is finally selected in the process of information generation. In a model using 'representation' as a holding structure, information change is reflected in the specification of the values (out of a possible range) in each of the dimensions.

'Mental representations' are thus pragmatic tools for handling information flow. Information in representations can be described by neurocomputational (e.g., connectionist) models (Rumelhart et al., 1987) (see description in the beginning of Chapter 2). We adopt a working assumption that representations are ultimately instantiated in brain neural networks (or cell assemblies) and correspond to subjective experience (see section 1.1.3). However, for our purpose, it is not necessary to demand detailed descriptions of brain neuron activities. We are not modelling neural events to exact details; we are considering brain-mind systems that employ an overall parallel distributed processing structure. We believe the structural characteristics of parallel distributed representations are relevant in providing a model that converges with some basic characteristics of subjective experiences (Dietrich, 2007; see Figure 2.5).

2.3.1 A neurocomputational account of mental representations

A simple neurocomputational (or parallel distributed processing, PDP) model is described here (see Figure 2.5) as a model for a basic mental representation for an external object.

The PDP model is inspired by the structure of brain cell assemblies. It consists of a number of processing units that are connected with one another through incoming, outgoing, as well as between-unit connections. At any time, each of the units can be either 'on' or 'off'. The on-off status of a unit is determined by the incoming signals. The unit receives weighted activation through connections from a number of other units, either in the same population of units or from a different population of units, or from sensors in contact with the environment. The incoming connection is active if the upstream unit is in an 'on' state at the previous time-step. The incoming activation then interacts with the 'weight' of the connection (or synapse) to produce an input to the receiving unit. The greater the weight, the more the influence of the incoming signal. From the different incoming lines, activations are summed up to produce a total input. The sum of all input then determines whether the receiving unit will subsequently be 'on' or 'off' according to an activation function (the activation function can be a step-threshold, a linear, a sigmoidal, or a probabilistic function). If the unit is 'on', its output line is activated and a signal is conveyed to the downstream units (see Figure 2.5).

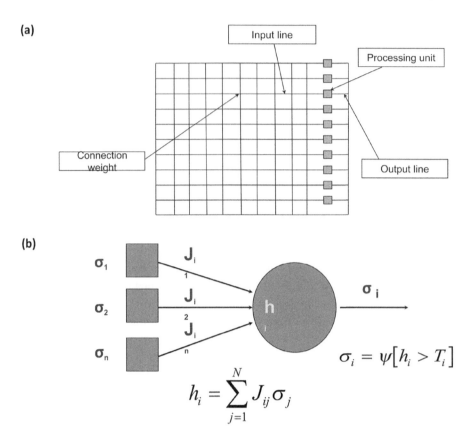

Figure 2.5. The parallel distributed processing (PDP) model. (a) An auto-associative network; the network consists of a number of 'neurons' (dark squares), which are the basic informa-tion processing units. At any moment in time, each neuron individually computes an output based on the input signal it has been receiving. The input signals are weighted by the connec-tion strength between the output axon of the upstream neuron and the receiving dendrite in the current neuron. The connection strength is modifiable according to past activity patterns (e.g., according to the Hebbian rule). In an auto-associative network, the output of the popu-lation of neurons feeds back to contribute to the input in the same population of neurons. Information is represented collectively in the activation pattern in a population of neurons. (b) Details of a computational neuron: σ: input value; J: connection weight. The summed weighted input (h) is fed into an activation function ψ, which then determines whether the neuron becomes activated σi; T: threshold for activation (see section 2.3.1).

This operation is computed individually for each unit at each time-step. Each unit therefore processes information in parallel to other units. In this model the representation is the pattern of activation across all units (distributed representation). Each unit may represent a feature (such as size, colour, shape, seats, doors, wheels), and the entire network may constitute a representation (such as a particular make of car e.g., an Austin Mini). The same architecture can store information about a number of different patterns (cars of different makes and models). The information is stored in the connection weights between units.

The network can learn to 'recognize' patterns if the synaptic weights can be modified according to the Hebbian rule (i.e., if the upstream neuron and the downstream neuron are both active at the same time, the weight between them is increased; Hebb, 1949). After learning exposures, the network can retrieve a pattern that it has 'encountered' before, even when only partial information of the pattern is presented. This ability enables content-addressable memory to be recalled based on presentation of partial contents, and not by specification of an address of the storage location. Content-addressable memory is a characteristic feature of human memory systems, in contrast to computer hard disk memory, which depends on a location address.

Uniquely, in contrast to classic mental representations, connectionist (PDP) representations can display 'graceful degradations'. If some of the many units constituting the representation are not functioning (or degraded), the network is initially able to compensate for the loss. This is because information about the memorized patterns is distributed over a large number of units and weights, and the mutual connection between these units can compensate for the loss of a few units. However, after a critical proportion of units have been inactivated, the memory function will eventually decline. Once it begins, the decline is steep. This dynamics of functional loss is consistent with clinicopathological observations in dementia. PDP models therefore exhibit behaviours converging with a number of clinical phenomena even without detailed modelling at the neuronal level (Dietrich, 2007). They also account for the mind's capacity to cope with noise and exceptions when processing is carried out by satisfying multiple soft constraints in a parallel fashion, in search for an optimal global solution, rather than via a rule-based algorithm. PDP models are particularly useful in modelling experiences such as memory retrieval, for example, the process of retrieving memory based on partial access to only part of the memory initially (content-addressable memory). In a PDP model, the initial information can trigger a snowballing process leading to the progressive retrieval of the entire pattern, via iterations of activation through relevant connection weights. These properties render PDP models well-suited to represent mental processes (Bechtel & Abrahamsen, 1991).

2.4 Evolutionary Perspective of Information Handling in the Brain

To understand the functions of the human brain from a biological perspective, it is important to have some ideas about the environment in which human brains evolved

(Crawford & Krebs, 1998). As evolution takes place across many generations over a lengthy time scale, it is necessary to inquire about the situation of human existence prior to recorded history. Despite a lack of written records, research in this area has furnished us with some ideas of what the human brain might have had to cope with in this early environment (Crawford, 1998). We postulate that selective pressure from this early environment should have contributed to shaping the human brain. This perspective can help us consider the type of information that the mind has originally evolved to handle in the original environment before the accelerated progression of human culture in the last ten millennia (Buller, 2006).

We expect that some features of the brain will still be adapted to the original environment. That environment however is unlikely to resemble the modern environment we live in, which has been transformed in many important ways over the last 10,000 years. It is generally assumed that the rate of emergence of significant new biological features in brain evolution is slower than changes in the environment. Adopting this perspective, we attempt to identify brain adaptations to the early environment with an awareness that some of these features may no longer be adaptive in the modern environment. Some features may even be considered as 'pathological'. The evolutionary approach thus offers insight into some scenarios that have arisen due to a mismatch between the brain and the rapidly changing modern environment. This kind of mismatch may not have to do with 'dysfunctions' in the brain itself. For example, in-built vigilance for small toxic animals and preference for high-energy food would have been adaptive in the early evolutionary environment but are less relevant in modern human life.

Current archaeological evidence suggests that several major transitions are relevant to our exploration (see Figure 2.6). In making inferences from an evolutionary perspective, we have to caution ourselves about the lack of details from earlier times and be open to revision in the light of new findings.

Before we contemplate the evolution of higher mental function in humans, it is important to acknowledge that some human mental-behavioural functions are shared with a wider range of species in the animal kingdom.

2.4.1 Mental functions in primates and other animals

An evolutionary approach has been adopted in the study of emotional expression. It was found that human facial expressions of some basic emotions are similar in other primate groups. Expressions and behaviour are consistently associated with the basic emotions not only for people from different cultures (fear, surprise, disgust, happy, sad, anger, pride, shame) but even across different primate species (anger, fear, excitement). Some of the emotions (e.g., fear) may be shared amongst an even wider group of animals.

Humans also share other basic behaviours with many animal species. They include sensorimotor functions, learning, fight-flight responses, seasonal changes in activity

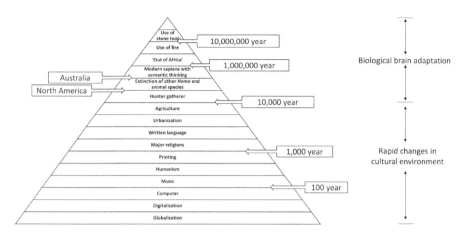

Figure 2.6. Major transformations in the human living environment relevant to the adaptations of the mind. Left of the pyramid: major geographical migration events; Right of the pyramid: estimated number of years ago; Inside the pyramid (from top to bottom): emergence of notable events. There has been an acceleration (increasing rate of change) in the transformative events.

levels, and dominance hierarchy behaviours (Cummins, 1996). Humans also share some higher cognitive functions with primates, who also have group living, reciprocal support, families, tribal wars, primitive tool use, and simple deception behaviours. However, other primates do not have the uniquely human capacity for syntax-based language (Goodall, 1986; Tomasello & Call, 1997).

2.4.2   Mental functions in early hominoid species

In the long period dating back over at least two million years, *Homo* species existed as intelligent 'pre-sapien' hominoid species, operating in smaller groups, capable of using simple tools, and becoming bipedal (Campbell, 1999). Paleontological evidence suggests that a number of hominoid groups coexisted in different territories. Social cooperation was vital as survival against larger and faster predators depended critically on group cooperation. Social exclusion would mean likely demise. Technological use of stone tools and of fire (Wynn, 1999) led to the practice of cooking food. The availability of cooked food may have contributed to a rapid increase in brain size (from 600 cc to 1400 cc), facilitating the emergence of *Homo sapiens* (see Figure 2.6) (Dunbar, 1998; Holloway, 1999).

2.4.3 Rapid mental development in *Homo sapiens*

The emergence of the 'modern human mind' is estimated to have occurred at least 100,000 years ago. Since that time, modern humans (*Homo sapiens*) have gradually spread to different continents. This process coincided with the disappearance of other hominoid species as well as the extinction of a large number of animal species. Modern humans appear to have emerged first in Africa and had then spread to other parts of the world, initially to the Eurasian land mass and then crossing the oceans to Australia (estimated 50,000 years ago) and to America (estimated 12,000 years ago). During the period, *Homo sapiens* lived mostly as hunter-gatherers.

Excavated artefacts from at least 30,000 years ago clearly suggest representational (symbolic) thinking, with the creation of novel representations consisting of artificial re-combinations of naturally occurring objects (Conkey, 1999) (see Figure 2.6). This development is probably associated with a snowballing increase in the complexity of human ideas, communication, and culture. Highly developed human language emerged as means to enhance group communication. Language based on universal grammar (syntax) allows complex propositional representation to be constructed for 'situational models', whether actual or imagined (see sections 2.2.1 and 2.3) (Zwaan & Radvansky, 1998). It enables symbolic thinking (Bickerton, 1995) and counterfactual thinking (Roese, 1994), as well as the passing on of complex technological and social information. Language also allows manipulations and deception, and facilitates the nuanced negotiation between cooperation and competition, within and between human groups (see section 2.4.3.1) (Franks & Rigby, 2005; Krebs, 1998).

Within human groups, cooperative behaviours can be considered from a perspective of survival (via various versions of reciprocal altruism) (Krebs, 1998). There was a need to detect 'cheaters' who took advantage of 'trust' within the group (Camerer, 2011). Language and gossip might have served important 'social brain' functions in these contexts (e.g., to communicate about the reputation of an individual, Dunbar, 1996).

It is not easy to appreciate the many unique features of human language because it is so proximal to our daily experience. One useful reflection is a comparison between human language and a computer programming language, which is designed for communication between man and machine. It can be seen that if the purpose were merely effective communication, it may not have been necessary for human language to acquire the many intriguing properties of flexibility, ambiguity, and context-dependence. Human language acquired these properties because language not only has evolved for communication but is involved in defining group membership, complex social negotiations, deception, and counter-deception roles.

2.4.3.1   *The evolution of human representational capacity*

It is important to consider cross-level interaction between physical, biological, and cultural information in evolution. Human ideas are sometimes constrained by biological factors. Both brain factors and genetic factors constrain ideas. For example, the dorsolateral prefrontal cortex imposes a limit to the maximum capacity of human working memory (Baddeley & Hitch, 1974; Miller, 1956). This limit constrains cognitive activities. For example, the maximum number of digits in a telephone number is limited by the human working memory span. Genetic constraint resides in preferences in the mind that are selected because they favour survival. One example is the preference for carbohydrates as a high-energy-value food source. In the evolutionary environment, food was generally scarce. The preference for food with high energy values would have helped biological survival. This preference has survived into the modern era, even though it may now be responsible for 'pathological' obesity (Higginson et al., 2016). The mismatch between evolved biological features of the brain adapted to the environment many thousand years ago and the modern human environment is expected to lead to tensions that may have implications for mental health. These phenomena have been explored in the disciplines of sociobiology and evolutionary psychology (Barkow et al., 1992; Dawkins, 1982; Wilson, 2012).

Evolution has conventionally been adopted as a working hypothesis in biology. We have adopted this hypothesis tentatively, noting that many details in human evolution are still missing. The evolution hypothesis is based on the availability of time. Given enough time, random variation will generate adaptive features by chance. Once an adaptive feature has occurred by chance, it is selected to persist through self-replication (see Figure 2.2).

Just as biological systems are open to the environment and evolve in adaptation to the environment, the evolution of ideas is shaped by pre-existing ideas in the individual mind and in the group (see Figure 2.2). Ideas interact with other ideas to produce meaning. Successful integration with other ideas facilitates the survival of ideas in individual minds and in groups (see section 2.2.3). Successful ideas may (though not necessarily) act to confer biological advantages.

For example, it has been speculated that at some stage in the course of hominoid evolution, the use of fire was incidentally discovered. The ability to use fire confers a number of advantages. This skill was transferred from generation to generation. The human brain has a high capacity for trans-generational transfer of cultural information (Rothbart & Posner, 2007). A necessary condition is the ability to communicate complex information.

A crucial step in human cognitive evolution involves the ability to use mental representation to conceive of objects and situations not immediately present in the environment (e.g., in tool-making, Uomini & Meyer, 2013). The human mind can entertain representations that do not concretely map onto existing objects in the external world. The capacity for generating such representations enables the contents of the mind to be freed from being bound by externally observable objects in the world. This pivotal capacity for human representations is indicated by the archaeological presence of imagined art forms as well as the use of symbolic processes in burials, rituals, and bodily decorations (which suggest the dissociation of representations from being bound by reality). The development of capacity for forming representations apart from those directly coupled with the external world was an important stage that heralded the emergence of a powerful representational system capable of handling complex ideas and intricate social relationships (Joordens et al., 2015).

One further aspect in the development of human language is worth noting. The tension between competition and cooperation within a group means that language evolves not only to serve cooperative communication but to serve competitive functions as well. The simultaneous need to serve both cooperative and competitive functions has resulted in the unique form of human language with its characteristic ambiguity (as opposed to the clarity in computer programming languages). With ambiguity, the possibility of deception multiplies (Noble, 2000). Deception implies a possibility for the betrayal of trust, which presupposes a state of 'trusting' and 'relating'. The fundamental place of trust and relating in human social interaction is supported by many empirical findings (Alós-Ferrer & Farolfi, 2019 [e.g., in Trust Games]).

It is proposed that the human mind fundamentally engages in 'relating'. The human mind has the propensity for relating to others, to nature, and to the Divine (Dessalles, 2000; Noble, 2000). Moreover, phenomenology of subjective experience suggests that 'relating' is a basic mode of operation in the human mind (see section 2.7).

2.4.4 Psychopathological insights from evolutionary perspectives

The human brain has acquired different layers of functions from different evolutionary periods. These functions can be broadly grouped as basic survival (fight-flight response), technological (empirical mastery of environment), social (primate group), and representational (complex ideas and relationships). Modern human activities have produced accelerated changes to the environment. Brain functions are adapted to an earlier environment. Biological brain evolution might not have caught up with the changes in the environment. Mismatch between the brain and the rapidly changing environment may be responsible for some mental distress and psychopathology.

2.5 Major Types of Information Handled in the Human Brain

2.5.1 Perceptual, environmental, social, and historical information

The brain has evolved to handle a diverse range of information. Different modes of computations are required for handling information for different needs. For example, depending on the interaction context, the brain may deploy interactional paradigm according to the complexity expected in the interaction (e.g., regular one-person game, two-person game, and complete randomness) (see section 2.5.1.3). The brain is expected to have developed distinctive modules to handle these different scenarios.

2.5.1.1 Instantaneous perceptual information

Perceptual information is processed by the brain to support moment-to-moment movements and actions (see Figure 2.7). This information is rapid, continuous, and transient. Being constantly updated, the information is directly linked to incoming sensory signals (bottom-up processes dominate).

2.5.1.2 Stable information about the physical environment

The fact that it is at all possible for Natural Science to discover rules suggests that there is a knowable regularity in the environment. Knowledge can be acquired through exploratory activities. Exploratory activity involves a sequence of actions coupled with predictions of environmental responses (Swenson & Turvey, 1991). Information is gained by comparing the brain's predictions with the actual responses from the environment. Deviations from the predictions provide information for revision of the prediction calculations. This revision process gradually shapes an emerging internal model of the target phenomena. Comparison of the actual response with the predicted response allows fine-tuning of the model. When exploratory learning has accumulated sufficient knowledge, the internal model makes increasingly accurate predictions that incrementally approximate the actual outcomes (see section 3.5.1). The ability to predict thus increases with time. This process is mediated by the dopamine system. Discrepancies between the internal model prediction and the reality initially trigger dopamine responses to facilitate further learning (Jensen et al., 2006; Talmi et al., 2013) (see Figure 2.7).

This interaction between the individual mind and the physical environment is a 'one-person game'. It involves one active agent interacting with a passive stable environment with hidden regularities. The ability to technically master a passive environment is an important aspect of the human mind. This 'technical brain' has probably developed to a high degree in early humans before the rapid evolution of the 'social brain'. It is interesting to note that psychopathological experiences such as delusions seldom only involve the interaction between the person and the physical environment.

2.5.1.3 Game-theoretic social information

In handling information related to interacting with others who are 'active agents', 'theory of mind' (TOM) and 'game-theoretic' representations are involved (Krause et al., 2012; Umeda et al., 2010). A game-theoretic framework considers 'others' as agents with intentions and strategies similar to oneself. Game theory addresses social transactions between two or more individuals. The participants are treated as equals in their ability

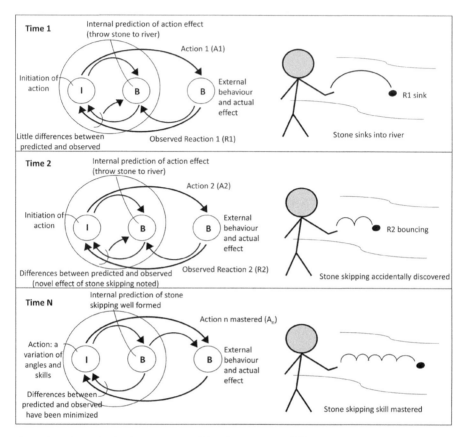

Figure 2.7. How the brain acquires stable information to 'fill' a representation about acting upon the physical environment (stone skipping). The process of enhancing the prediction accuracy through repeated comparison between predictions and observed outcomes is illustrated in the figure. We use the example of stone skipping (or stone skimming). As shown in Time 1 and Time 2, the skill is learnt through fine-tuning the angle and strength of the throwing action after observing the differences between predicted reaction and observed reaction. Actions that lead to the intended outcome are reinforced (remembered so that future repetition is more likely). In a series of explorations with variations in the action (angles, torque, strengths), the action is incrementally tuned to reduce the difference between the predicted and the actual outcome. The skill is mastered when the differences between predicted and observed outcome have been minimized. When this happens the mental representation (internal model) for stone skipping is 'filled' (see section 2.5.1.2).

to think of the best strategy. The 'game' typically leads to different outcomes depending on the selected behaviour of each of the participants. Game theory models then ask what might be the optimal strategy for a participant. Games can be 'cooperative', in which participants need to cooperate to win together. They can also be 'competitive', in which participants win at the expense of others. Strategies are markedly different in competitive games compared to cooperative games. In real life, both competitive and cooperative elements are present in social interactions, often at the same time. In addition, others are never entirely predictable (see section 5.3 on empathy) (Colman, 2013). This presents a challenge fundamentally different from the one-person game (see section 2.5.1.2), which involves one-way interaction with a passive physical environment. In social relations, predictions do not enjoy the same certainty as in the physical world (see Figure 2.9). This is the realm where intentions and ongoing revisions of probabilities are required. The nature of uncertainty involved in this situation is not just one of measurement errors but of guessing intentions and of predicting behaviours in others (O'Brien et al., 1998; Tomasello et al., 2005). Others can be competitors who act deliberately in an unpredictable manner. Most delusions involve contents that are social in nature. Errors in representing others are prominent in delusional states.

2.5.1.4 *Historical, veridical information*

Possible 'future states', after having transited into the past with the passage of time, become 'past states' committed in memory. In the future, there are many potential States of Affairs (SOAs) (see Figure 2.8). In contrast, in the past, there is usually only a single version of events that prevails in autobiographical (historical) memory (see Figure 2.8). Historical memory refers to events that have taken place; the memory is usually shared. There is also individual (private) historical memory when the experience does not involve others.

2.5.2 Tentative situational models in the human mind

The most challenging type of information for the human mind to handle is information about possible future situations and uncertain current situations. Propositional language is an information container well-suited for formulating interpersonal scenarios about the current SOA. SOAs have a tentative nature that is not present in perceptual information handling (Dietrich, 2007). This tentativeness is important as several competing hypotheses are often entertained at the same time. During the period of deliberation, further information can be reviewed before the closure of an interpretation. This minimizes the risk of premature conclusions (see section 2.5.1.3). This capacity is illustrated by a classic detective story plot. In the opening, the initial scenario sets the context (e.g., the crime scene), leading to a number of possible culprits. The opening corresponds to a state of low information as a large number of possibilities remain. The detective then engages in uncovering additional information. Each piece of information

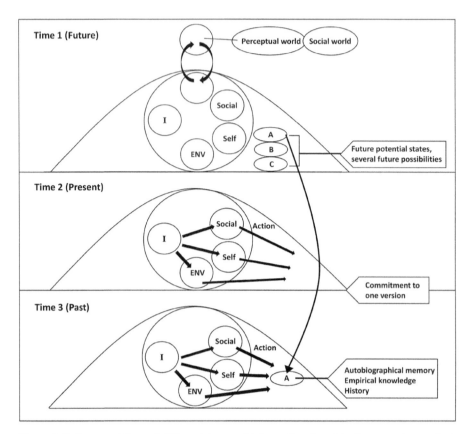

Figure 2.8. Temporal flow of different types of information in subjective experience. Each momentary experience consists of the following components: the active self, the experienced self, the physical environment, and others, each of which are experienced through mental representations. Mental representations are informed by interaction with the world through perception and action. In addition to pointing towards the current objects, mental representations can point to future and past objects. In Time 1, the centre circle represents current experience at Time 1, consisting of mental representations for the following components: I, social, self, and environment, which interact with the perceptual and the social world; the circles on the right are mental representations for potential future states, depicting several different future possibilities A, B, and C. In Time 2, in the centre circle, 'I' creates actions on social, self, and environment and has thereby become committed to one of the previous possible future potential states (A, from Time 1). In Time 3, the committed future potential state (A) contributes to information in autobiography, empirical knowledge, and history (see section 2.5.2).

will alter the probability of a particular suspect as the final culprit. Eventually a critical piece of evidence emerges and resolves previous dilemmas, narrowing down the suspects to just one and solving the crime. The identification of a single final culprit corresponds to a state of high information. During the process, it is important for the brain to be able to keep open the files of possible suspects and to revise probabilities associated with different suspects in an ongoing manner. In a detective narrative, the initial evidence often leads to a high probability being attributed to a wrong suspect. The classic detective plot is engaging exactly because it invokes a 'natural' processing mode of the mind. This leads to a drive for information in the readers' mind. This information is fed incrementally by the writer. The reader will be misled when the ability to 'keep the files opened' is compromised. Consequences of premature conclusions can be appreciated in delusional experiences in which the tentativeness of the SOA is 'collapsed' to the concreteness of perceptual certainty.

In handling highly complex probabilistic information, the human brain has developed a capacity to tolerate uncertainty instead of concluding with the closest solution (as in confabulation, Moscovitch, 1995). This ability maintains a space for holding back from the most immediate (dominant) interpretation. The toleration of uncertainty enables an opportunity to entertain alternatives and allows the possibility for revision. This space however is costly to the mind as it requires the simultaneous holding of multiple SOAs (see section 2.5.4) (Zwaan & Radvansky, 1998). As this ability to hold, to compare, and to monitor a number of tentative options is demanding on computational resources, pathological conditions may compromise this capacity. Inability to hold this tentative deliberation space open may contribute to the formation of delusions and delusion-like ideas. Delusions are notoriously difficult to define. It is noteworthy that amongst the different characteristic features of delusions, the inability to consider alternative accounts may be the closest to being a 'defining feature' (Jaspers, 1913/1963).

2.5.3 Fractionation of streams of information

Information transfer involves changing the SOAs (i.e., situational model) in the recipients' minds (Zwaan & Radvansky, 1998). Information transmitted via discourses (see Figure 6.3) is used to specify objects and the relationships between them in the situational model. Accurate social information keeps the receiver's inner 'model of the world' updated and relevant. Accurate mental representations of other people allow an individual to be effective in relationships.

Synchronization with the environment takes place continuously in real time. In contrast to synchronization with the physical movements, where fast perceptual information is handled, in social situations, a slower and a more tentative process handles more complex information. It is likely that the brain utilizes two different systems for the computation of (1) fast and clear signals and (2) slow and ambiguous signals (Kahneman, 2011). Whether the appropriate channel (fast or slow) is activated for a given context can be of significance in psychopathology.

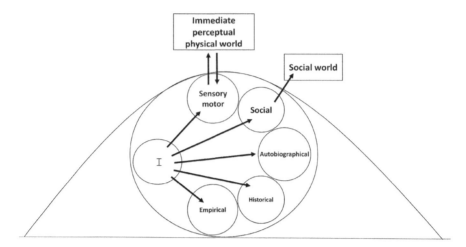

Figure 2.9. Different domains of information are involved in subjective experience. Inside the circle (from left to right): mental representations for 'I', 'me', sensory motor, social, autobiographical, historical, and empirical domains; mental representations interact and are informed by the outside world (outside the circle), consisting of the immediate perceptual physical world and the social world (see section 2.5.3).

We can also make the distinction between information that is for temporary usage, such as perceptual details in particular situations, and information that is preserved and accumulated over one's lifetime (see Figure 2.9). The former type of information is less relevant for the long term and is not retained by the brain. For the latter, there is a global accumulation of information over time for the individual, with a possibility of transferring to a group (cultural) platform. Within a given experience, information from a number of different levels is simultaneously encountered, from perceptual levels to semantic levels. To enable different modes of processing, information is likely to be extracted and processed separately at the different levels (Shapley, 2004; Ts'o & Roe, 2004) (see section 6.6).

2.6 Information Exchange in Human Groups

In a group, the individual can be considered as an information unit for which information is a 'currency' (similar to material resources such as food) that can be used in transactions.

Exchange of social and technical information is one of the key processes in human transactions (Dunbar, 1996). A piece of information may contain a 'value' as determined by its 'social significance'. The human mind has a disposition to search for salient social information (Barkow et al., 1992). Social significance results in a change in the situational model in an individual, in such a way that the individual re-positions his social network configurations adaptively to guide his future social actions.

Information therefore is valuable if it is of value in guiding such positioning to social actions. Valued information is often novel, timely, and consequential for the reordering of social configuration in the situational models. Significant novel information spontaneously engages the mind. Recycled or redundant information is not engaging. Judgement of the value of a particular piece of information for 'others' is an important aspect of TOM (Astington & Jenkins, 1995; Dunbar, 1996).

Social information is continuously updated. Exchange of social information is an important mechanism for managing social group memberships. Individuals in a group are identified by shared information. They also use social information as a currency in cooperative and competitive interactions.

The mind is endowed with an in-built capacity to receive information presented in accordance with the structure of human narratives. Human language has a universal structure (Pinker, 1994/2010). A sentence unit is constructed from three basic components: the subject, the action verb, and the object (see Figure 2.10). This structure is 'propositional'. The same structure can be filled with different contents. It has been

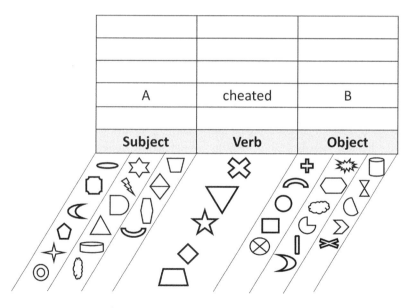

Figure 2.10. Propositional structure as representations. Complex representations have a propositional structure. A propositional structure is 'language-like'. The structure links a subject and an object with an action (verb). For example: A (subject) cheated (verb) B (object). Each of these positions can be filled by alternative mental objects, represented by the different shapes. Each of the positions can either be a simple elementary object or it can be a proposition itself, embedding within itself a subject, an object, and an action (see section 2.6).

proposed that this predicate-argument structure has evolved in the human mind to represent social relationships (Worden, 1998).

With this representation, humans move beyond constructing knowledge of just the material world (one-player game). They start to compose situational models of their social worlds (multiplayer games; Colman, 2013). The capacities for empathy (see Chapter 5) and TOM (Astington & Jenkins, 1995) are essential products in this process.

Social information is continuously updated. Exchange of social information is an important mechanism for managing social group memberships (Noble, 2000). Individuals in a group are identified by shared information. They also use social information as a currency in cooperative and competitive interactions, such as defending against deception (Knight, 1998). Irrelevant information is filtered. Redundancy is steeply curtailed, so that only individuals with within-group shared background information (context) can fully appreciate a specific piece of information. Individuals consume energy to actively search for high-quality information.

Members in possession of valuable information are trusted and valued within the group. The mind is continuously searching for salient information. The brain's salience system makes comparisons between the presented information and known regularities. This comparison enables the detection of novel patterns. The mind also examines new information for internal coherence and for consistency with existing schema in its semantic net. Reconfiguration is carried out by the mind to minimize incongruity. This process results in the re-organization of long-term memory.

What constitutes a group? How large are human groups? What are their boundaries? What defines the relationships between different groups? The size of a human group in the prehistoric era has been estimated to be just over one hundred. In modern society, groups are much larger and far more complex. There are also more interactions between different human groups. Groups are defined by shared common purpose or identity. Group identities in the modern world are often conceptual in nature, as contrasted with historic groups, which may be more ethnic and genetic.

There are tensions between the information that enhances agreement in a local group and the information that aligns a local group with a broader range of groups. The openness to a broader range of widely accepted 'reality' is an important function. Without reference to a broader 'reality', excessive alignment exclusively in the interest of local agreements may lead to unchecked distortions within a smaller group. As a result, there is a need for some 'fidelity' to a broader 'reality' in a larger group to counterbalance the self-perpetuating tendency to agree within a smaller group. Failure in this process leads to 'groupthink' (Janis, 1982).

The social nature of the human brain enables an appreciation as to why distorted mental representation of other people is a frequently encountered content in psychopathology.

2.7 Information and the Relational Nature of Human Experience

For mankind, information is not only used for adaptive utility. Indeed 'experiencing' itself can be of primary value in human life.

Recognition, sharing, and exchanges of experience are primary driving forces in human social life. Many messages in social communication testify to this: 'My experiences are well perceived by my friends', 'my friends are envious of my travel experiences', 'I have the unique fortune to experience this in my life.' It can be said for many people that 'our experiences define us'. We are unique as individuals in our experiences. For the reason that experiences are unique, they can be meaningfully shared. It is evident that in modern society, experiences themselves are increasingly being sought after in human transactions (see section 4.3, the experience economy, Pine & Gilmore, 2011). Shared information is of value not only for adaptive actions but also for defining the individual within a group. Thus, one's experience enables one to construct a mode of 'existing in relation' (see section 3.5). 'To relate' is to impart information to 'other' minds so that there is a possibility for the sharing of experience via language and imagination.

2.7.1 Beyond information: Towards a concept of health

At the level of a population, more information does not necessarily lead to a more 'desirable' progress. To define what is 'desirable' involves value judgements. We shall pragmatically consider a 'desirable' direction as one that leads to increased 'wholeness and growth possibilities' in individuals. This also implies a direction for the attaining of optimal 'relating' between the individual human mind, nature, and other human beings.

It is important to recognize that a high-information state may not necessarily constitute a desirable direction indicative of progress. A high level of organization can be present in a narrowly focused, self-seeking direction that eventually leads to maladaptive outcomes. Recent history of mankind has demonstrated that this scenario has been involved in a number of historical catastrophes (Harari, 2011/2014; Yu, 1988). In these tragic situations, one tell-tale sign is the restriction in the possibility of 'relating openly' to other minds, to nature, and to the Divine (Boyer, 2000).

'To relate' means 'to communicate'. To communicate is to impart new information to another person's mind and to receive new information openly from another person. In a narrow sense, to increase information means to convey specific information to reduce the potential possibilities in others' minds. Relating is thus mutual. In the process, I become 'understood' (or 'specified', associated with a higher information state) in your mind, and at the same time you become 'understood' in my mind. However, in communication there is a possibility of not only specifying information in given dimensions but also creating a new information space. This space is creatively formed with 'relating'. Information interacts between the semantic worlds of the participants and can become meaningful in new ways in their minds. Mutually acknowledged information becomes the background for further creative explorations. In this way, a network of interacting growth paths linking individuals is enabled. Relating to other people in an authentic way is an important condition for individual growth.

The notion of 'openness in relating' as a 'desirable direction' is related to the idea of 'health'. Health is conceptualized as a state of 'well-being' in physical, mental, and spiritual dimensions (World Health Organization, 1948). The idea of 'well-being' is not a fully definable end state but a direction for a continuing aspiration. Of note, 'unhealthy' paths can also be highly organized sometimes. If the increase in information is for self-seeking, it can eventually lead to a *cul-de-sac*. Apart from information, health leads to openness to possibilities, growth, and harmony in relating on a broad front. It is not narrowly self-seeking and may indeed involve self-sacrifice. On the other hand, unhealthy growth directions often lead to less openness and a narrower focus. It is perhaps easier to conceptualize unhealthiness as leading to an increasingly narrow path in the way a person engages his Lifeworld.

The view of health being related to openness converges with the idea of homeostasis in biological systems. In health, biological systems are maintained in a stable equilibrium (i.e., homeostasis: an internal state regulated against perturbations in the environment). Negative feedback systems detect small perturbations and initiate mechanisms to restore homeostasis. In contrast, positive feedback systems respond in such a way as to reinforce perturbations, leading to escalations in the original change. Such one-way systems lead to instability and are seldom encountered in nature. Similarly, for the mind, if a situation leads to further and further escalation of the original changes along a narrow path, we should be alerted. While homeostasis is a necessary criterion when considering health, it is on its own not sufficient. A stable system may be free from disease, but it may not necessarily be considered as being in a state of positive health.

The state of health for the individual mind and for human culture inevitably touches upon "relating". We have now seen that information can be factual, technical, social, and relational. It is important to further explore the relational properties of the human mind (Lock & Symes, 1999).

2.7.2 'Being in relation' as a fundamental human experience

The range of human mental activity is broad; a cursory survey reveals many activities that point beyond immediate biological survival. For example, aesthetic experience is preferentially facilitated in conditions that are not constrained by functional needs. Freedom from functional demands enables the making of a genuine choice. This is a precondition for actions that are associated with aesthetic experiences. 'Choosing' involves a freedom to align with more 'sublime' principles that operate beyond concerns of immediate functional needs. Aesthetic activities are primarily about making choices in a manner that can inspire others. These activities are therefore primarily relational.

Aesthetic experiences are important for human identity. Aesthetic capacity (i.e., a person's propensity to be aesthetically inspired by a certain information) is relatively personalized. Capacity for aesthetic experience is therefore associated with a sense of identity. Being able to respond aesthetically to some aspects of the world engenders a sense of belonging to life. In the experience, one allows oneself to resonate deeply with higher realms beyond oneself.

When the light of aesthetic experience illuminates us, it invites a child-like joy. One is called to relate to something greater in life, to belong and to be grateful. It carries meaning beyond narrow mundane calculations. Such inspirational experience produces an alignment with life that often is valued as an ultimate 'meaning' (Maslow, 1943). Such moments bring us closer to the experience of the divine. It elicits in us a response that can be more open, more trusting, and more accepting of contradictions. This state of mind inspires us towards the ideals of 'well-being' (Ananth, 2008).

Relating in real life is often mundane. Handling tensions and incongruities involving "others" is a skill a developing person needs to master (failures may underlie maladaptive social behaviours). Tensions are resolved, for example, by re-configuring some representations or by selectively refraining from accessing some information. The manner in which this internal tension is handled is a measure of inner consonance of the mind (Abelson et al., 1968). Failure to integrate and resolve tension in internal representations results in difficulties in adaptation (e.g., in dissociative conditions) (Festinger, 1962).

In the 'inspired' mode, inner tensions subside through subjugating diverse representations to alignment in one dominant direction, which point to something larger and beyond. This alignment can offer hope when it is experienced beyond the chaos and disorders of daily encounters. Inspired moments of aesthetic experiences are capable of transporting one into a more sublime mode of existence.

In summary, we started with inquiring about the functions of the human brain. We considered the central role of the brain in information handling. We revisited the ideas that arise from an evolutionary perspective for the emergence of the mind, with its technological, social, and representational layers of functions. We have come to appreciate that non-material, informational entities need to be addressed not only in human science but also in biology. We proposed that the brain handles information with representations. This basic function of the brain lays the grounds for human experience. We shall consider the structure of subjective experience in the next chapter. At the same time, reflection on the nature of information also raises an awareness of the basic action of 'relating'. 'To be' involves 'to exist in relation'. 'To exist in relation' includes living in relation to others, to nature, and to the divine. The primary role of 'relating' converges with insights we obtain from phenomenological exploration of human subjective experience. This broad perspective of the human brain points to a fresh approach to psychopathological experiences.

3

The Structure of Subjective Experience

In this chapter, we shall explore the structure of subjective experience from the perspective of 'the one who is experiencing', examining information that is directly accessible to us as raw experiences. Having consolidated a biological background to the handling of information by representations in the human brain, we now switch to consider our experiences 'from within', using phenomenological explorations.

3.1 Introduction to a Phenomenological Perspective

Phenomenology studies subjective experiences from the perspective of the experiencing person. The word 'phenomena' refers to how experiential contents appear to our minds. We shall keep to a minimalist account with phenomenology. We start with the absolute minimum and build up our model only when an additional feature is required. We begin with a simple phenomenological stance from the early phenomenological circle, adopting a position that does not challenge the notion that the external world has an existence independent of our minds (realism). A minimalist approach is essential to ensure that we do not add to the model in an unconstrained manner.

The key processes we shall visit are as follows: We start with the most essential components of subjective experience—I (as the subject) being aware of (the action) me (the object). I, the subject, also relate to other objects and states of affairs (intentionality). Some objects and states of affairs are located in the real objective world (realism). I also relate to 'others' as experiencing agents similar to myself (empathy). The objects and states of affairs are representations. Apart from pointing to what they represent, they are also mutually connected in a semantic network. Life experience consists of a continuous process in which a person's potentiality unfolds into actualization through action. Actions can be self-determined and creative.

3.2 *Cogito Sum* as the Starting Point of Phenomenology

Phenomenology does not use empirical science as the starting point. Instead, it sets out from its own foundation in 'primary experience'. Phenomenology uses our direct experience 'as starting points for understanding ourselves and our world' (Brentano, 1874/1973; Husserl, 1913, 1921/1970). In this way, it strives to construct a broader view on human knowing. From the phenomenological perspective, scientific knowledge is only a special kind of knowing (Stein, 1916/1970, 1931/1998).

3.2.1 *Cogito sum* as the minimalist starting point

The most irreducible fact that we are immediately certain of is the fact of our own being. Thinkers throughout the ages had utilized this starting point (e.g., St. Augustine of Hippo, AD 400/2012, Descartes, 1644/1983, and Husserl, 1913, 1921/1970).

Compared to '*cogito ergo sum*' [I think, therefore I am] (Descartes, 1644/1983), phenomenology starts with an even simpler '*cogito sum*' [I think, I am]—that is, I am, and I am aware of this being with an unreflective certainty that precedes our rational knowledge (thus not yet involving a reasoning process involving the 'therefore') (Stein, 1916/1970). *Hence there is no need for the 'ergo'. 'Cogito sum' is a necessary and sufficient starting point.*

3.2.2 The three basic components of *cogito sum*

The starting point of *cogito sum* involves three fundamental components (see Figure 3.1):

1. The 'I' that is the acting 'self'.
2. The 'me' that I am aware of.
3. This act wherein I am aware of myself ('I' relating to 'me').

This minimalist starting position of *cogito sum* already implies a temporal structure. William James (1890) pointed out that the 'observing I' and the 'observed me' are located on a time continuum, and the current 'I' observed the 'me' a moment ago (see Figure 3.1). Relating and temporality are thus fundamental aspects of human experience inherent in this starting point (Stein, 1916/1970).

3.3 Temporality of Human Experience

A fundamental feature of human existence is the fact that we can exist fully only in the present moment. The present is sandwiched between the future and the past (see Figure 2.8). Human experience is a continuous flowing of experience from the future to the past.

However, 'what was but is no more' and 'what will be but is not yet' are not simply nothing. Past states and future states are not simply 'non-beings'. The transitory nature of human experience renders it a unique mode of existence, spanning time with a gradient of 'existence' with different intensities (Stein, 1916/1970).

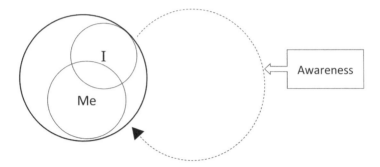

Figure 3.1. The three minimal components of *cogito sum*. Inside the left circle: 'I' and 'Me'. Right: awareness, which takes time. The 'I' is the active experiencing agent of the self, and the 'me' is the 'self' as experienced by the 'I'.

3.3.1 The present moment

The present moment stretches backwards and forwards (see Figure 2.8). Importantly, it is only in the present that a person can make choices and act on the world. This unique character of the present moment has been appreciated in many traditions (Hnat Hanh, 1967; Sahn, 1976). For example, mindfulness practices encourage individuals to focus on the present moment and be detached from the past and the future (Hnat Hanh, 1991; Kabat-Zinn, 1990).

3.4 Atomic Unit of Experience

3.4.1 The atomic unit of experience: *Cogito sum*

We construct a model of human subjective experience by starting with the basic unit of experience, *cogito sum*. This minimalist model consists of the following components: (1) the reflecting 'I' as the subject, (2) awareness of 'me' as the object, and (3) the act of awareness (see section 3.2.2). In this process, time is inherently involved. The 'me over time' is involved as both the object and the subject. As the process of awareness takes time, the 'me' that I am aware of is the 'me' a moment ago (see Figure 3.2). Thus the basic unit of experience contains (1) the 'I' now, (2) the 'me' just past, and (3) a temporal sequence (Stein, 1916/1970).

These components are knitted together in time into an evolving whole that constitutes the stream of human experience. The past, the present and the future are entrained into a stream of consciousness (SOC) (see Figure 3.3).

Potentials (i.e., possibilities) are inherent in this basic human existence, as the present holds potentials for the future (see Figure 2.8). The change in information state over the passage of time is a fundamental aspect of human experience (future

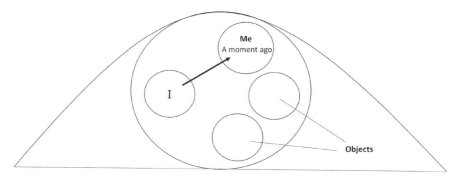

Figure 3.2. The atomic model of experience: *Cogito sum*. 'I' acts on 'me' a moment ago (see section 3.4.1). The 'I' relates to the 'me' through the act of awareness (not reasoning, hence Decartes' 'ergo' is not in Stein's *'cogito sum'*). This process of relating is a core aspect of experience. The process of awareness takes finite time. The 'I' is aware of the 'me' a moment ago. Time is thus also a core component of experience (see section 3.2.2).

possibilities become past certainty; see section 2.2). *The notion of 'information' is therefore inherent in the temporal nature of human existence* (see section 6.5.1).

The present moment is a moment of contact in a unit of continual passing. In the passage of time, potential becomes actual, moving progressively out of the future and into the past (see Figure 3.3). Mankind is always progressing in transition. Human 'being' can therefore be considered as being in a process of 'becoming' (Stein, 1916/1970).

The stream of consciousness (SOC) is weaved together by a string of atomic units of experience (see section 3.4.1 and Figure 3.2).

3.4.2 The structure of momentary experience units

In the present moment, the unit reaches the height of being (see Figure 3.3). The content of this experience consists of the intentional object, the intentional act, and the experiencing 'self' (Stein, 1916/1970). The 'self' is like a vessel, transient and holding the content of experience from moment to moment (see Figure 3.3).

3.4.3 Objects in the atomic experience units

The objects (or things, *rerum*) being experienced are organized into semantic categories. Some of the objects are 'real' objects and are appreciable to others in the external world. Others are 'possible' objects and are only sharable to varying degrees.

'Objects' are grouped in the mind into categories. Categories are organized hierarchically or as a network (as in the semantic network) (Rosch, 1973, 1975). Objects can belong to a general category or be an individual exemplar, or both at the same time

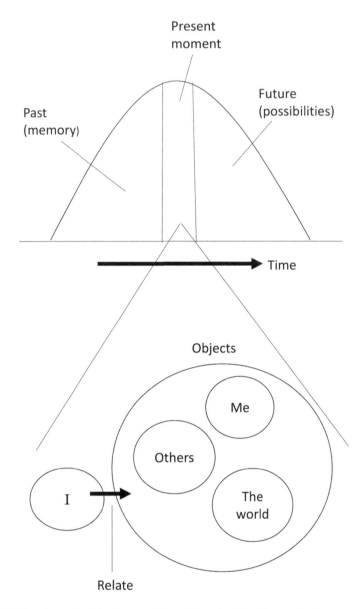

Figure 3.3. Structure of subjective experience. Time includes the past with memory of past events, and the future with possibilities. In the present moment, 'I' relates to objects including me, Others, and the world (see section 3.4.2). Experiences of the past and the future share a continuity with the present. However, the 'I' can only act on the external world in the present moment.

(see section 6.2). 'Objects' in the mind are handled as representations (see Figure 2.3). Complex representations of a number of objects organized in a propositional relationship are 'states of affairs' (SOA, see section 2.5.3). The mind also relates to SOAs. It is important to understand that the mind in fact interacts with the world through mental representations rather than 'directly' making contact with the outside world (see section 2.3 on representation).

3.5 Convergence: The 'Relational' (Intentional) Nature of Human Experience

A fundamental nature of the subjective 'self' is that it does not exist in isolation. It always exists in relation to 'something' else. One of the primary properties of the mind is *to relate* (see Figure 3.4 and section 2.7).

This intrinsic nature of the self as 'relating to' and 'pointing to' objects is very important as it highlights the fundamental essence of the self as existing in relation to something other than itself (see section 2.7.1). Thus, the self in its very nature operates in the mode of going beyond 'itself' (relating to something else). In fact, developmentally the individual is probably aware of the external world earlier than he becomes aware of the 'self' (see Tomasello & Call, 1997; Tomasello et al., 2005). In this process, the 'awareness of self' can also be considered as becoming aware of oneself as part of the 'external world' (Card, 1998). The relative positions of the 'self' differ in different cultures. In collective cultures such as the oriental culture, less weight is placed on the individual 'self' compared to the 'community'.

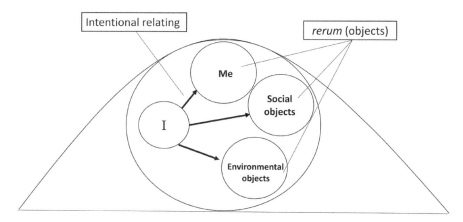

Figure 3.4. The 'intentional' (pointing) nature of the human mind. 'I' is intentionally relating to rerum (objects). Objects include the self as 'me', others as 'social objects', and the physical world as 'environmental objects' (see section 3.5). The pointing relationship between the experiencing agent and the objects of experiences is a fundamental feature of subjective experience.

3.5.1 Relating and information

There have been studies about the ways in which one can relate (mental acts) to mental objects (representations). Early phenomenologists made a distinction between a 'presentation' mode of relating and a 'meaning' mode of relating (Pfander, 1900). In the 'meaning' mode, the object is engaged in a conceptual act; it is related to other semantic concepts and is often not elaborated in its perceptual details (as expressed in the saying 'the rose is gone, the name remains', Eco, 1980/1983). In the presentation mode, the object is engaged in a perceptual and non-conceptual manner, and intuitive contents (perceptual details) can be fulfilled (Reinach, 1921/1969). It is possible that the two ways of relating are mediated by different brain systems (Dietrich, 2007). Ritzel (1916) pointed out that meaning acts and presentation acts are different because they point to different objects. Meaning points more to semantic concepts (as objects) while presentation points more to external objects.

Relating can also be viewed from a dynamic perspective. With experience, the details of an object can be enriched through repeated exposure. The primary mental action of relating can be described as a progressive process of knowing. We shall first describe the simpler process of relating to a passive physical object. First there is an 'awareness of the presence' of an external object. This is followed by a process of exploratory interaction leading to gradual acquisition of information about the object. Eventually when relevant information about the object is totally acquired, a 'complete grasp' (mastery) of the object is attained (Skinner, 1938; Stein, 1931/1998). When this happens, the object can be 'left' to 'be related to autonomously' in the mind of the subject. This state is reached by gradual exploration. The mind utilizes an internal model to predict the external object's response. If the actual response is different from the prediction, the model is revised. The revision continues until a good predictability is achieved. Learning consists of iterative filling of the representation by interaction with the object in the real world (see section 2.5.1). After the object is thoroughly explored, its representation becomes 'full', and the object becomes predictable (see Figure 3.5). The process will then be allotted less attentional resources. Exploration is facilitated by motivational drives. Before achieving complete mastery, partial predictability constitutes a strong drive for further exploration. Information itself becomes a primary reward in this partial reinforcement situation (see section 2.5.1.2) (Skinner, 1938). Thus the human mind is driven towards the 'filling' of external objects by progressive mastery. This simple description depicts the 'relating' to a physical object. In relating to another person, the interaction is more complex. The two participants mutually influence one another. Each of the participants is at the same time knowing and being known (see section 2.7).

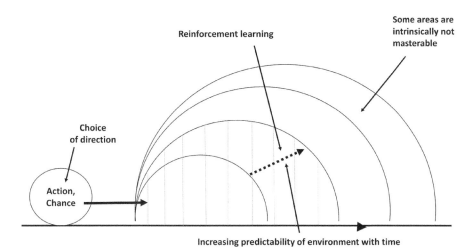

Figure 3.5. Increasing mastery of the environment as expansion of predictability in the world. As time goes, the environment is increasingly becoming more predictable as learning takes place. However, it is important to recognize that some areas in the environment are intrinsically not masterable (see section 3.5.1).

4

Unfolding Phenomenological Processes in the Human Person

4.1 Engaging with Life Experiences

After considering the basic unit of experience (see section 3.4.1), the act of experiencing (see section 3.5), and the objects of the experience (see section 3.4.3), we now turn to a broader perspective to consider the Person as the living agent that is acting and experiencing in his Lifeworld throughout time.

In the psychopathological assessment, the Person is often considered as a passive recipient of 'life events' and other stressful 'factors', with scanty considerations of his active role in his Lifeworld. This bias had arisen from a narrow perspective of the Person.

We propose a more comprehensive account of the individual's active interaction with his world. This view emphasizes (1) a development path leading to the individual in his present circumstance and (2) the individual can make active choices regarding his development path. Psychopathological conditions impact how the individual makes active choices in his Lifeworld. The engagement of a subject with his Lifeworld involves the specific engagements with his own physical body as well as with objects in his proximal environment. When a person relates to his world in a creative fashion, objects that he relates to are animated and 'imbibed with life'. Understanding the roles played by the active person is important for clinical assessment and management.

The life development of a person can be considered as a process of 'actualization' that involves the unfolding of potentials with time (Stein, 1931/1998). It is useful to consider each life experience as engaging the person in some specific domains. Stein (1931/1998) described an 'interface with life' in which the person contacts each external object and life circumstances at some prescribed 'levels'. Engagement with life experience leads to accommodation and assimilation in the mental model, resulting in a gain in information. Before the encounter, the potential for knowledge is referred to as *Intellectus possibilis* (possible insight) (see Figure 4.1). This is a potential that can only be fulfilled with future encounters. After a successful encounter, new knowledge emerges. *Intellectus possibilis* is transformed into 'habituality' as the individual masters the new knowledge. In this process, information is created in the person's mind as fulfilled representations. As a result of biological potentials, active choices, and life opportunities, the person develops unique 'habit structures' with fulfilled representations.

Habit structures then enable behaviours that further influence the cascades of engagements in subsequent life encounters.

Some people choose to engage very deeply with some aspects of life. Others
choose to engage more superficially. It is possible to live one's life with only superficial
engagements. If there is only minimal engagement, the deeper layers of potentiality in
a person remain latent and not actualized. This is a situation that has been described as
inauthentic living (Macquarrie, 1972).

Some limits to the potential in a person have already been laid down from the
beginning of their life. The unfolding of that given potential eventually depends on
personal choice and circumstances (see Figure 4.1). The engagement process changes
what is in the external world as well as what is in the inner world. When potentials are
not actualized, opportunities in both worlds (internal and external) remain unfulfilled.
What is not actualized is lost forever. The loss is not only in external opportunities but
also in the unfolding of that person's potential, in that their actualization is less than
what could have been. The actualization of individual potentials as fully as possible
through proper engagement is an important aspiration in human life.

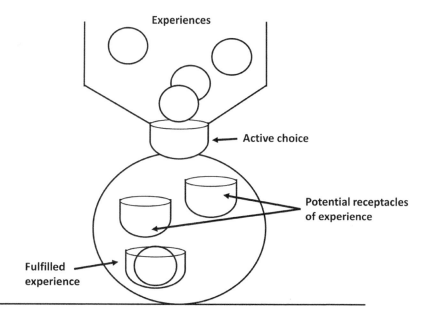

Figure 4.1. Engagement of a person with potential experiences. A person has some degree of
choice over engaging with different experiences in life. Potential experiences (opportunities)
are represented as circles. The person has some degree of choice in selecting the experiences for further processing. The person's capacity to receive experiences is represented by
empty receptacles. There is individual variation in capacity to receive experiences. Once the
experience is engaged, information is obtained, it becomes a fulfilled experience. This is represented by the circle being engaged in one of the potential receptacles, I (see section 4.1).

Once at a Chinese tea shop, the owner was having a conversation with an elderly Buddhist nun. After a good infusion of fine tea, the owner laid out the tea leaves and said, 'After producing a good cup of tea, these tea leaves have fulfilled their missions in life.' The nun said, 'It is indeed important to live as these tea leaves; many people today are not engaging their full potentials. Many are paralysed by a false sense of modesty; others are plagued by a lack of self-confidence. One should aim to fulfil one's potentials and make good use of one's gifts in life, no more, no less. It is not a matter of responsibility; it is a matter of natural development.' For patients with psychiatric conditions, stigma would make this struggle significantly harder. A key role of the clinician is to support patients in the development of their full potentials, minimizing the impacts of the illness.

4.1.1 Potentials for the reception of experience

Humans show individual variations in their abilities to fruitfully engage with specific aspects of experience. Conceptual capacities are required to master specific areas. For example, the ability to engage with advanced mathematics is not endowed with every person.

In learning, there is a transition from potency to action, from the 'possible' to the 'realized'. In this process, information is generated. After learning, the mind is more 'specified' than before (see section 3.5 on information).

Some areas of experience are pivotal, in that engagement with them will lead to the mastery of a 'seed' structure (mega-representation) that can be of use in a number of other areas. In this way, new areas can be more easily mastered after the 'seed' structure is attained through hard work in the initial area. One example is traditional Chinese calligraphy. Through calligraphy, one acquires a sense for the oriental aesthetics of movement and stillness, space and foreground, subtlety and force. These aesthetic principles generalize to other oriental artistic domains, such as music and poetry. It is not surprising that oriental arts are often considered as a set (e.g., music, Go, calligraphy, and painting). Similar functions have been suggested in the learning of Latin in European education. The language provides a 'seed' structure for organizing experiences. Clinicians should have a broad knowledge of the various life domains even though they themselves may not be able to engage with all of them. In this way, they can appreciate the pattern of Lifeworld engagements and developments in their patients.

4.1.2 Experiences and meaning

Individual background shapes the reception of life experiences (see Figure 4.1). Incoming information interacts with existing information in the mind. In this interaction, existing knowledge templates accommodate the incoming information. Existing templates are already organized within an individual mind to produce an optimal degree of coherence. The degrees of fit between the incoming information and the pre-existing knowledge structure determine the 'meaning' of the information. When the fit is insufficient, there is difficulty in making sense of the incoming information and the individual needs to decide whether to wait or to explore more. If the fit between the incoming and the existing information is high, the incoming data do not confer much additional information. The experience is redundant (consider the repetitive uneventful journeys between work and home).

When learning has occurred, an experience is mastered. The experience is associated with a 'fulfilled' representation that the mind can use to predict future responses. The representation of the fulfilled object becomes assimilated into the individual's world (Piaget & Inhelder, 1969) and the phenomena become largely predictable.

Evaluation of how a person engages with his Lifeworld is of primary concern in psychopathological assessment. Engagement at different levels of life activities defines the developmental path of the person. Engagement is a progressive process of mastery in different life domains. Importantly, the evaluation of how a person engages or not engages with various life domains can give important information about the factors that have determined his path. This evaluation will inform not only a person's capacity but also about his choices.

4.2 Choice and Agency

The 'I' engages life experiences as an active agent in experiencing the Lifeworld. In the present moment, the 'I' can decide whether to engage with a particular aspect of the Lifeworld. Although the decision is suggested by positive or negative dispositions, these factors can be overridden. Ultimately, the 'I' can make decisions counter to these factors.

4.2.1 Motivation and preferences

Humans manifest positive and negative dispositions towards objects (*rerum*) in his Lifeworld. These dispositions prompt the individual to engage or not engage with particular aspects of the Lifeworld (in an act of choice). The mental world of an individual develops according to these choices. Nevertheless, individuals have the freedom to finally decide whether to follow the preferences.

4.2.2 Choice and freedom

At the present moment, and only at the present moment, the subject 'I' can make a choice over the *direction of engagement* with life. The selection of the direction of engagement will result in the building up of his Lifeworld in a particular direction. This choice narrows down possibilities. With increasing engagement and the selection of a specific path, more 'information' is incorporated into the experiential trajectory of an individual. In this sense, the path that the subject has chosen to follow is a creative work of art, a path carved out by his choices.

There is a saying that 'we make our decisions, and then our decisions turn around and make us' (e.g., Brandom, 1979). Like it or not, each person is an artist, creating his own life through these choices. It is true that some have easier material to work with than others, but there is usually some room for creative decisions. When clinicians encounter a patient, they see a person *and his artwork*. Likewise, patients see both the person and the artwork in the clinicians too.

4.2.2.1 *Choices in everyday life*

Much of daily decisions in life is about maintaining a freedom of choice (or at least an apparent freedom of choice). Individuals act to avoid being cornered into a situation where life experiences are largely forced upon them by external circumstances (Klyubin et al., 2008). Even a dichotomous choice is cherished as better than no choice.

In the modern digital world, apparent choice is flourishing. In contrast to the material world, where physical resources are limited, in the digital world experiences can be multiplied easily. An increasing variety of commodities offer a large number of 'choices'. In real life, much of an individual's effort is consumed in maintaining a state in which as much choice as possible is available. Thus in shopping, in vacation, or in food, the consumer marketing world often capitalizes on 'a sense of having choice'. In the modern era, the initiation of a new activity is often engaging (as there is a perception of choice to start something new) whereas persistence in a sustained direction is often more difficult (where less choice is perceived, in comparison to starting a new direction).

Passive choice involves choosing amongst several options. This is common in consumer activities such as shopping or dining. In contrast, creativity involves creating new space for action. An intermediate form between creativity and passive choice is the selection of options from alternatives in a larger set of slots in a given structure, in order to generate a novel re-combination. The Japanese tea ceremony is an example. In the tea ceremony the occasion is individualized by choice in the flower presented, the tea bowl chosen, the calligraphy displayed, and so forth, which is unique and unrepeatable for each occasion.

Choice gives one a sense of agency and individuality. Making a choice involves a narrowing down of possibilities. Choice is therefore directly linked to information (see section 2.3 on information).

In supporting recovery from mental disorders, offering as much choice as possible is a widely used strategy. Extreme deprivation in everyday individual choices occurs in the setting of large institutions and has been explored in the phenomena of 'institutionalization'. It is important to distinguish between the various levels of creativity involved (passive choosing and more creative choices). It is an empirical question whether creative actions are better than passive choice in facilitating recovery.

4.2.3 Habitus as a product of cumulative choices

With the passage of time, the potentials in a person become more or less actualized in reality. The individual's developmental path often involves physical objects. The set of material assets (*habitus or proximal environment*) a person acquired and selected throughout his life can become somewhat 'animated' objects. Even the person himself can become an 'animate artefact' (a product of human creative activity). The person, his acquired objects, and the living environment surrounding him are shaped by the cumulative decisions of the person (see Figure 4.1). For example, the set of 'accessories' belonging to a person reflects his creative preferences. Some explicit examples are personal libraries and collections.

4.2.3.1 *Animated objects*

Beloved objects are 'ensheathed with forms' from the owner's mind. Such animated objects belong to the non-material 'realm of the spirit'. These animated objects are closely connected with the mental life of the owner (such as a teapot, a pen, or a book). By being closely linked to human activity, objects 'come alive' in an 'animated' world. They offer more through their 'forms', rather than in their materials, and are received into *the life stream of animated beings*. The term 'life stream' refers to the sphere of interaction between living beings over time. A material object can acquire a living relationship with a living agent. A house that has been inhabited for long enough, a book that has been read and re-read, a cup in hand day after day can all have a spiritual dimension. They exist in relation to a mind. In this regard, a good clinician always learns from the *habitus* of patients, which provides important cues over the life choices of the individual. Keen observation akin to detective work is required for astute psychopathological investigations.

4.2.3.2 *How 'predetermined' is the developmental path of a person?*

We have discussed the role of individual choice in determining a developmental trajectory. However, there are also suggestions that development unfolds for an individual according to some predetermined pathways. Is the development path determined at the outset prior to development or is the path not fully predetermined but unfolds only during the actual development process? Empirical discrimination between these two alternatives is difficult because of the never-retraced nature and uniqueness of each moment in an individual's life. This fact limits the possibility of repeated empirical observations under controlled conditions. We have therefore adopted a pragmatic position rather than an empirical position on this matter.

4.2.3.3 *Creative actions of the mind*

In creative activities, things (*rerum*) are reconstituted from existing materials. Materials are never created from nothing by human action. When the object becomes an artefact, human ideas 'live' in the object, and through this object meanings are communicated to others (Stein, 1931/1998). Meaning is intrinsic to the act of creativity.

The 'spirit', as opposed to substance, refers to the animated, non-material aspect of human existence. Creative activities produce information in an animated realm. The 'spirit' derives information directly from the 'spiritual' world (Hegel, 1807/1977), by engaging in an animated interpersonal information flow.

The oldest surviving forms of such human creation are cave paintings (Conkey, 1999). They can be considered as marking the dawn of the human ability to use symbols as inner constructs in the mind that are not directly bound by the immediate environment (Wynn, 1999).

The study of creativity is a *via regia* in investigating the generation of information. In producing creative objects, the mind/brain performs its most distinctive roles (Andrieu, 2006). It re-arranges material objects in its world in order to facilitate biological survival. In this process, objects become ensheathed with human information and become 'meaning-ful'. Shared representations are also handled as objects in human communities. The mind operates in a semantic world that is 'given' to humankind as only partially completed, leaving potential spaces that remain to be filled through creative actions.

A number of artists showing signs of mental health challenges have left collections of artwork (painting, prose, or music). Pondering over artwork by persons suffering from a mental condition can reveal something about the impacts of illness on their information-generating activities. In visual art it is not difficult to appreciate the cognitive signatures, for example, the high degree of repetition as well as the difficulties with proportions and spacing. These characteristics are related to cognitive changes in patients as a consequence of their illnesses (see artwork in Andreoli, 1996).

The creative interaction of the human mind with other human minds is a particularly interesting possibility. Empathy is the key process involved in this interaction. There are two senses of creativity in personal interactions. Creativity could mean the selection from a number of alternatives. This act of choosing generates information. An example is expressing your opinions to your friend, so that information is increased in their representations about you. Creativity at another level involves generating new potentials and new possibilities. These possibilities did not exist previously. In this act a new information space is created. Example for this may be inventing a new game or a novel group activity; individuals can then choose options in this new space to express themselves.

We can receive information through 'relating' authentically to other people (see section 9.6.3 on alignment in dialogue). We can choose either to be open or to be closed to such information flow. When we are closed, we treat other people as material objects. When we are open, we treat others as authentic, animated (spiritual) beings (Buber, 1925/1937).

The human mind dwells in a shared world that provides a context for individual creative actions. Creative actions are related to one another, through a network of common *experiential-meaning contexts*. Sets of creative acts contribute meanings to each other in this shared context (Stein, 1916/1970).

4.2.3.4 *Impacts of mental illness on creative actions*

In *mental illness* the intelligibility of the mental life of the affected individual can be compromised to the extent that it is no longer understandable (Jaspers, 1913/1963; Stein, 1916/1970). In some cases, the specific disruption of the *neurocognitive* processes corresponding to the physiological machinery of the brain (functional architecture) may produce discrete low-level disturbances in the mind without affecting the core of the person. However, in many types of mental illnesses, for example, psychotic disorders, higher level processes of 'relating' and 'meaning' are also disrupted. Processes impacting on the core of the person are thus distinguishable from processes that only affect isolated low-level modules of the mind (i.e., functional architecture; see section 1.1.1). Interestingly, this distinction was made more than a century ago by Wernicke (1881/2005). In the recovery from mental illness, creativity can play two roles. Firstly, making sense of the illness experience may require an openness to accommodate different experiences. Secondly, in neurocognitive function, the ability to switch contexts and to generate new items (divergent thinking) are important for the flexibility in handling life situations in the recovery process.

4.3 The Fullness of Experience in Health and Illness

Mental conditions, like physical illnesses involving severe pain, encroach upon the space for individual experience (Andrieu, 2006). Experience is reduced to an impoverished form. In distress, many subtle shades of the experiential space are omitted (resulting in a reduced number of feature dimensions in the representations). This reduction of feature dimensions is likely to occur in mental illnesses (mood disorder, psychosis, dementia, etc.). Compromised experiential space may also occur when under distress.

Mindfulness practices aim to restore the fullness of experience. Aesthetic 'peak' experiences produce similar effects. Rich experiential filling of the psychological space is not enjoyed by many people in many of their life experiences. It is something one may attain mostly only during vacations, upon meditative practices, or during reflective moments.

Phenomenologically rich experiences are important for mental health. In contrast, a compromised form of constricted experience is curtailed by stress or illness. One may conceive of mental health as an ideal state that engages with as full an experiential space as possible. The pressure of life in today's complex societies makes this ideal increasingly difficult to achieve.

In addition, in the absence of a purposeful direction in life, the state of experiential fullness may still be insufficient on its own. One psychological adaptation for modern sapiens is the 'story' (see section 8.5 on narratives), as expressed throughout history in dramas and literature. Through immersion in narratives, humans derive a sense of following a story with its anticipations, tensions, and resolutions. This is in contrast to the uneventful daily experiences in modern sapiens' life, which are specialized, narrow, flat, and deprived of the 'extremes' that nowadays occur literally only in 'dramas' in the entertainment industry. Exposure to the extremes of experience helps to 'orthogonalize the vectors' (see section 6.6) of experiential representations (Amit, 1989; Földiák, 2002).

Does this mean that sensational and diversified experiences are more valuable? In monastic life, one seeks simplicity and abstinence from material attachments. In doing so the consequences are twofold. There is the inconvenience of cold, hunger, and insecurity, which compromise the fullness of experience. In exchange, there is the freedom from the excesses of material abundance. This freedom facilitates high-quality experience. This aspiration is also in concert with the ideals of the oriental scholars aspiring towards simplicity and engagements with nature.

The richness of life depends on a right level of engagement with the external Lifeworld. Either too much or too little external engagement compromises the phenomenological richness of life experience (see sections 1.2.1 and 1.2.2). A lack of direction in life can render colourful experiential content boring and not meaningful, leading to a deliberate search for rewarding experiences as an end in itself. Such pursuit of an experience as an end in itself is common in the modern world and drives much of the economy of consumerism (e.g., the 'experience economy', Pine & Gilmore, 2011).

4.4 The Person and the Body

In the concluding part of this chapter we turn our attention back to the physical body of the self. It is through the experience of our bodies that we begin our experiences of other people.

The phenomenological experience of 'I' is intimately bound by an implicit experience with 'my body'. Experiences are presented to the mind through the tangible body (e.g., in feeling a table). The body has fields of sensation and can be spatially located in the perceptual field of the sense organs (Stein, 1916/1970). Biological changes in the body are also experienced in specific and direct ways (e.g., adolescence or menopause). As the mind operates within the body, it can be described as an 'embodied mind'. The body is a 'given' condition in our experience. We are bound to our body in specific ways. For example, our visual world is referenced from a first-person spatial location of the perceiving 'I'. This visuospatial reference frame has a specific point of origin, a 'zero point of orientation' located somewhere in the head (Stein, 1916/1970). We have a 'self-centred' visual space. Importantly, the body can be experienced simultaneously in a twofold manner: (1) as a first person directly receiving bodily sensations and (2) a third person body as one of the objects in the world, being perceived from the outside (Card, 1998). Confluence between these perspectives during self-initiated movement is essential to the sense of agency (and through this to the sense of self). Discrepancies may contribute to anomalous experiences such as the delusion of passivity.

Through our living bodies, we can experience the world in 'lively' (animated) manners beyond the direct senses. For example, when we see a table, we do not only passively perceive the visual pixels of the table. We also 'sense' its other attributes such as its texture through touch. This 'filling-in' of experience is 'given' to us through 'top-down' processes in our mind. Likewise, in active manual exploration of an object, our own hand movement is integrated with the resulting sensation. Our experience is the sum total of the contact with the table, integrating the tactile information from our hand with the hand's dynamic actions. These layers of experiences are embedded within one another as an integrated complex. The experience includes cascades of 'if-then' components (i.e., if I move in this manner then I should feel this). This 'if-then' cascade of prediction is intrinsic to our exploration of a given environment. Importantly, such exploratory cascades are also involved in the empathic perception of a living person just as in the exploration of the physical environment. In my mind, I can imagine my movement without actual bodily movements. Similarly, it is possible to explore the perceived mental state of a person through 'empathic intuitions' (see section 5.2.1). It is important to recognize that my mental explorations of the physical and human objects are nevertheless bound by my own body schema and my own mental attributes, respectively.

4.5 Representing the Body and Representing Others

What permits other people to be perceived is firstly the awareness that they appear to have bodies similar to our own. Another person's living body is appreciated as another centre of orientation but in the same spatial world as our own. Another 'zero point of orientation' apart from my own is in existence in the same physical space. This recognition is the beginning of empathy (Stein, 1916/1970).

Through empathy we can access another person's orientation system and through this we can reflect back on our own position. We can then be aware that our own point of reference (spatial and psychological) is only one amongst many. In this way, we are no longer bound by our own self-centric perspectives and can go beyond our individual world 'as appearing to me only'. Empathy enables us to break through these boundaries. It is only by acknowledging the presence of others that an appreciation of an 'objectively real' outside world is possible. Empathy is thus a precondition of objective knowledge of the external world.

Even though the person is located in a 'centre' of awareness that experiences his Lifeworld, he does not have the breadth nor time to personally engage with the entire world. The world is much larger than can possibly be fully engaged in a single individual and his lifetime. The person also does not have the intellectual potential to engage with all the different kinds of possible knowledge in the world.

The individual path of a person in his engagement with life must therefore involve choices in the narrowing of options regarding his engagement with different possible facets of life. Some experience of his world will therefore be 'second-hand' and built upon his ability to construct his experience based upon other people's knowledge.

5

Empathic Access to Other People

Our discourse so far has largely focused on the relationship between mankind and external objects. These objects are truly 'external' (empirically external objects, EEO, Kant, 1781/1998) only if they can also be observed as such by other minds. Importantly, this condition presupposes our ability to appreciate other minds (Stein, 1916/1970). This capacity is empathy. Empathy is central to the phenomenology of real-world experiences. In this sense, 'the external world' is inherently communal.

5.1 Representing Others and the Phenomenon of Empathy

Husserl (1913, 1921/1970) emphasized the engagement of the mind with EEOs as a fundamental aspect of experience. However, the world consists not only of physical objects but also of other experiencing agents just like ourselves. 'Others' are therefore presented (see sections 5.2.1 and 5.3.1) to us not only as physical bodies but also as animated bodies with sensitivity. Like us, others are constituted from material physical bodies and non-material minds. We come to acknowledge that others can not only confront the world in similar ways as we do but also communicate with us, treating us as objects in their world (see section 4.1.1).

The mind engages 'others' through empathic processes. Empathy broadly refers to processes where information from the object's (others') mental state generates a mental state in the subject that is more applicable to the object's mental state or situation than to the subject's own prior state or situation (Preston & De Waal, 2002). Empathy includes a range of emotional, cognitive, and behavioural phenomena such as emotional contagion, sympathy, cognitive empathy, and helping behaviour. Empirical observations from psychology, ethology, and neuroscience suggest that some empathic processes are even shareable across different species. They also show effects of familiarity, past experience, and cue salience. Empathic processes can be parsimoniously handled with a perception-action model, which emphasizes the shared use of the same representation between incoming perceptual information (about the other) and outgoing action planning (of the self, Preston & De Waal, 2002). The perception-action model has received empirical support through the discovery of mirror neuron systems in the brain (di Pelligrino et al., 1992).

Lipps (1903) was the first to propose a mechanistic account for empathy (einfühlung, translated to English as empathy by Titchener (1909)) by suggesting that the direct observation of emotional gestures and expressions in others will prompt the motor mimicry and the brain activation patterns associated with the same emotional expressions. Similarly, McDougall (1908) proposed that sympathy involves the activation of instincts based on the perception of bodily expressions in other people. Meltzoff (1994) observed that infants can imitate the facial expression of others. He proposed that humans can derive information about others' emotional states through the association between their own emotional states and facial expressions. While such 'simulation' theories account for low-level empathic phenomena such as shared emotion, the understanding of higher level empathic processes such as motivations, desires, and beliefs may require additional processes. For high-level empathic processes Mill's (1893) inference from analogy is recognized as being inadequate and the use of folk psychology in mentalizing others' intentions has been proposed. However, folk psychology mind-reading theories mostly address high-level intentions in empathy. It appears that an essential aspect of empathy, namely the sharing of raw experiences, has been relatively poorly addressed. While empathic communication of raw experiences may not be a common activity in everyday life, it is crucial for psychopathological evaluation. Access to raw subjective experience is the primary concern in the phenomenological tradition. Phenomenologists such as Stein and Husserl have treated empathy as an irreducible experiential act *sui generis* (Stein, 1916/1970).

Stein used a phenomenology framework to analyse and describe the various processes related to the phenomena of empathy. She not only emphasized the bodily aspect of empathy but also discussed the cognitive aspects of the phenomena of trying to understand the mental state of another person. This account is coherent with our initiative to construct an approach that addresses the processes whereby anomalous subjective experiences can be clarified and communicated in psychopathological assessments.

One particular process involved in the access to the mental state of the 'other' involves the active use of explorative processes (action and thoughts) to explore the potential state in the 'other'. This can be attained through interaction, applying past knowledge, and the use of internal simulation using a model of the 'other' (theory of mind). This process has been termed 'empathic explication'. The process is similar to the active exploration of a physical object. It also involves 'top-down' processes (see section 5.1.2).

5.1.1 Primordial quality of experiences

The first question is whether emphatic processes are 'primordial' phenomena. Perception is about sensing in the physical world. Sensations come to us as concrete experiences bound to our body and constrained by our sensory organs. This constitutes the everyday experience of physical objects in the 'external world'. This experience is concrete and direct and is considered as 'primordial'.

The close coupling of sensory perceptions with bodily sense organs is the basis for some illusory perceptions. In these illusions, the experience is still primordial (Stein, 1916/1970). For example, in the well-known Müller-Lyer illusion, two lines of equal length were perceived to be longer and shorter due to outward-pointing and inward-pointing arrows at their ends, respectively. This illusion is a genuine subjective phenomenon. The underlying mechanism involves our visual system in the brain, which utilizes built-in angle detectors in judging distances and sizes.

In contrast to active choice and agency, some of our experiences are imposed upon us and are not the results of our choices. They are important constituents of our experiences. The occurrence of events out of our expectations is a 'fundamental given' in the human condition. These unexpected events are essential to the awareness that an objective world exists apart from our intentions (Jaspers, 1913/1963).

Perception of external objects is associated with a belief that the objects will continue to exist regardless of whether we continue our perceiving act. In this sense an external object is contrasted with objects of imagination and memory. This concept of object permanence (Piaget & Inhelder, 1969) is important for drawing a boundary between imaginations and hallucinations. Imageries are not primordial: Although they are vivid, they are also perceived as being under our voluntary control. Hence they are recognized as internally generated phenomena. On the other hand, hallucinations do not require our continuing efforts to sustain them.

An important phenomenological feature of memory is that we can recall memory contents *at will*. In healthy subjects, even though one cannot control the exact content of memory association, it is possible to control the direction of the association. In exercising this control, we are managing the contents that can be present in our conscious awareness. This control is compromised in some mental conditions, resulting in the intrusion of unwanted contents into conscious awareness (e.g., obsessive-compulsive disorder and post-traumatic stress disorder).

Experiences of imagination and memory are to varying degrees 'depleted' of the vividness of real perception. Jaspers (1913/1963) describes these experiences as lacking in 'substantiality'.

Empathic experiences are similar to memory or imagery and different from perception in that they involve appreciating the perspectives of a person to whom we do not have direct sensory access and are not bound to the sense organs (e.g., eyes). They also involve our use of 'top-down' knowledge, as well as ongoing 'explorations', to grasp a more 'all-rounded' appreciation of the other person.

5.1.2   Empathic explication

Experience of physical objects can be subjected to extended mental (and physical) exploration (feeling the texture, exploring the unobserved visual aspects of an object, etc.). Empathy for the mental state of another person involves similar processes. This process can be called 'empathic explication' (Stein, 1916/1970). In the perception of physical objects, explication corresponds to physically exploring the different facets of an object to obtain more complete information (e.g., by looking around, feeling around, opening and closing, handling in different ways). This is a closely coupled interaction between our exploratory action, perception, and the unfolding information about the object.

Explication is a process that we have already learnt to use to different extents. For instance, in exploring an object with a complex shape based on a two-dimensional photograph, we fill in the gaps where we do not have direct information. How we fill in the three-dimensional model depends on explication. We can mentally play with possibilities. For example, what if I turn the object to the left on this occasion? What happens if I view from the top? Studies have revealed details of how the mind 'rotates' a mental image just as if it were a physical object (Zacks, 2008). Based on available information and anticipation we can usually do quite well in filling in the unknown. For the more experienced, mental explications can be carried out for complex tasks, for example, in musicians rehearsing a piece of music without the instrument or in physicists imagining the outcome of a 'thought experiment'.

Empathic explication is an important process in the clarification of psychopathological experiences. When we come to explicate another person, we employ empathy to allow us to 'feel' the mental state of the other person; we continuously explore through further interaction to obtain additional information and to check the accuracy of our model. In empathic explication, during clarification of a symptom, iterations of questions are asked to fill the feature dimensions in the representation for the symptom.

5.1.3 Non-primordial nature of empathy

How can the experience of another person be 'given' to me? It cannot be through *directly* experiencing the same experience (this would have been telepathy). Empathy is possible through my trying to receive this through efforts that involve an active reaching out from myself (actively receiving the experiences of the other person through communication) and an active reception of this reaching out (the other person willing to be accessed). The experience of empathy has some 'as if' qualities of imagination (e.g., in its being subjected to voluntary control).

As we do not directly access another person's experiences, individuals are truly separate. Individual experiences are not directly connected (a failure in recognizing this perhaps is encountered in ideas of reference in the psychotic state). The acknowledgement of this boundary between individuals is part of authentic empathy. Empathy recognizes that access into another person's conscious experience is only partial. Paradoxically, as a result of this recognition, the other person becomes less illusionary and more real.

5.1.4 Phenomenal characters of empathy and memory

Our experience of empathy is not as concrete as perception (i.e., primordial), just as our experience of memory is not primordial. The act of empathy is closer to an act of remembering than an act of perception.

Our experience of memory is a reduced form of less intense perceptual experience (e.g., *The name of the rose*, 'the rose is gone, the name remains', Eco, 1980/1983). Memory becomes an internalized representation and is available to our voluntary manipulation and recall.

The memory of a joyful moment is about experiencing 'the memory' of the joy but not 'primordial' with respect to experiencing the joy itself. The content of the memory (the joy) is not primordially re-experienced but is 'embedded' in the experience of the 'memory of the joy' (we shall call this an 'embedding' process).

Current non-primordial representations may point to past primordial representations. The past is a former 'now'. In the transition from a primordial to a non-primordial experience, the representation becomes less vivid and more open to manipulation.

When the 'present I' engages the 'past I', it was the 'past I' that experienced the joy. The content of memory is not primordial. Personal memory may be construed as an empathic process initiated from the 'present I' towards the 'past I'. That is, the 'present I' tries to appreciate what the 'past I' had experienced. However, the 'present I' cannot directly re-live that experience. This awareness is key to the psychopathological assessment, as often we inquire the 'present I' in the patient about the mental state of the 'past I' who experienced the symptom in the past (see section 9.3.2.2 on clinical dialogue). The experience retrieved by the 'present I' about the symptom is an embedded representation. The 'present I' does not directly re-experience the past experience. The experience is embedded in memory of the 'past I' (see section 9.3.2.8).

Similarly, the content of empathy, that is, the experience of 'the other' ('foreign subject'), is 'embedded' and not primordial, just like the contents of memory. It is an experience that is covered with layers of embedding. These layers of embedding make empathy non-primordial (Stein, 1916/1970). In psychopathology, it is necessary to appreciate the existence of these layers of packaging in which the original experience of the patients is embedded (see section 9.3.2.2 on clinical dialogue).

5.1.5 Limits of empathic experience

We understand other people's experiences through empathy. Empathy allows us to contact other people as persons, as agents similar to ourselves. Importantly, in this way empathy also lays the foundation for objective knowledge of the external world (see Chapter 1). The affirmation of other people's ability to experience the external world constitutes the basis for 'objectivity' (i.e., objectivity is by definition that part of our experience that we believe can be shared and verified by other people). From the phenomenological perspective, empathy is a foundational experience that enables the objective knowing of the external world, as well as a subjective knowing of another person's experiences.

The intelligibility of the other person is bounded by our own experiential structure. Our capacity to empathize is ultimately limited by our own personal experiential and knowledge structures. Individual experiential structure may determine the extent to which people can optimally engage empathetically with one another. In oriental wisdom there is an ancient saying: 'how can one fathom the mind of a gentleman using the heart of a mean person'. Putting aside the moral connotation, the limitation in understanding another mind with one's own has been recognized by the ancients. Clinicians can enrich their experience of people through interaction with different people socially, as well as through engagement in cultural and literary experiences.

5.1.6 Significance of empathy for the person

Empathy is central to the constitution of the human person. In empathic relations we secure the basis for acknowledging other individuals as 'beings like myself'. With empathy we can see the world from others' perspective and see ourselves as others see us. In this way we can appreciate that our own perspective is but one of many. In this awareness we are fully constituted as persons. Through the awareness of other people, the world can become independent of our consciousness. We are able to see it as unlocked from a self-centric perspective (see Figure 5.1). To understand 'my

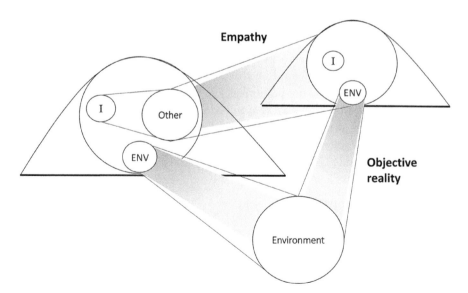

Figure 5.1. The roles of empathy. With empathy, we understand that others have their own views on the environment. This awareness that others may see the environment that we are also seeing is fundamental to the sense of objectivity (see section 5.1.6).

world', 'others' are essential. In this shared Lifeworld, we can communicate with others through a common system of symbols and meanings.

5.2 Shared Meaning in Subjective Experience

5.2.1 Mutuality in semantic representations

Information is continuously being acquired from the social and physical environment to update an ongoing semantic system in the individual. This is a system whereby a large amount of interconnected information interacts to enable construction of a coherent whole (Solé et al., 2010). These connections exist beyond the direct mapping of some semantic symbols (words) to the outside world. The mutual inner-connections engendered possibilities of new meanings that arise as a result of internal intersections. Within these new possibilities lies the root for creativity. We may note that the generation of a new level of meaning is dependent not only on the amount of information but also on the possibility that the information interacts between themselves to produce a new level of emergent meanings.

Through mutual support of meanings in ideas, individuals not only share symbols that map to the world as external anchors, they also share an internal world based on consistent relationships between these externally anchored ideas. This sharing presupposes that these internal semantic maps are also somewhat consistent between individuals. The inner semantic world of different individuals contains nodes that are constrained mutually by the shared external symbols and their relationships. Importantly, even though they are not directly linked to shared external referents, individuals can often communicate using these symbols meaningfully, as if they also map onto a shared internal meaning space. Individuals do share to some extent a collective inner world. Some ideas can have no external reference and can still be shareable across individuals. In some cultures, they are shared knowingly (as in legends and myths). In this case even though they do not correspond to the 'real' concrete world of external reality, they are known to be located in the shared imagination (e.g., as a myth) and distinguishable from the external reality.

To summarize, experiential information can be located in the following domains in the mind: (1) individual subjective experience (private); (2) individual-shared subjective experience through empathic communication (shared); (3) shared subjective experience that maps to culture but does not map to the external world (cultural); and (4) shared experience mapped to the external world (empirical).

In psychosis there is often a breakdown of boundaries between these different domains.

5.2.2 Homeostasis of individual models of reality

The vital process of maintaining an updated and accurate model of the world is assured by a continuous interaction between the individual semantic world and the real world (see Figure 5.2). Discrepancy between the real world and its semantic representation leads to a disequilibrium that is normally handled by assimilation and accommodation processes in the mind (Piaget & Inhelder, 1969). In assimilation the new information is incorporated to enrich existing structures in the mind. In accommodation, existing structures are modified to respond to the new information.

If the mind fails to assimilate or accommodate, a lasting unresolved misalignment between the inner semantic world and the outer reality may emerge. This may lead to difficulties in relating to other people.

5.2.3 Interaction between representations and 'reality'

Individuals communicate with others in their real world primarily through dialogues. Significantly they also use inner speech with 'their representation of others in their mind' to 'rehearse' a conversation. This inner modelling process generates predictions that are then compared with empirical results when they are encountered in real

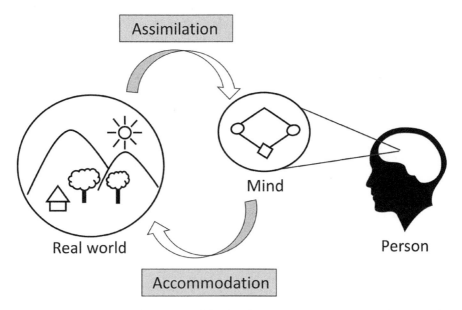

Figure 5.2. Homeostasis of mental models of reality. A continuous interaction between the individual mental representations and the empirical external world is maintained through ongoing processes of assimilation and accommodation. This leads to a managed correspondence between the mental models and the empirical external world (see section 5.2.2).

dialogues with the person (Bayer & Glimcher, 2005; Corlett et al., 2007; Holroyd & Coles, 2002; Schultz, 2007).

In this way individuals adjust their inner representations of others according to feedback from real-world interactions, until they attain a good match between the representation and the external situation. Unlike the mastery of physical objects, mastery of others as 'animated' objects presents an inherent degree of unpredictability. This is implied by a game-theoretic consideration: when two persons interact, it may be in their interest not to be totally predictable to the other person (two-person games, Colman, 2013). The interactions with persons should therefore engage the mind in a different mode (social, two- or multi-person game) from the interactions with the environment (physical, one-person game).

5.2.4 Representation of 'reality' in psychosis

When a psychotic experience occurs, anomalous judgements of reality result in misalignment between self-representation and the representation of others. This results in a disequilibrium in the representation system that cannot be resolved except by deriving further anomalous interpretations.

The following positions summarize consequences of an anomalous experience 'A' (e.g., a hallucination):

(1) I believe that others are as real as me.
(2) I think my experience A is real (as it is primordially experienced).
(3) I observe that others do not think A is real.

If (2) and (3) have to be confronted, some reason has to be generated to account for the difference. These reasons can lead to secondary delusions (e.g., others are influenced by some powerful forces or others are not who they are) (see Figure 5.3).

5.3 Representation of Reality in a Group

We can extend the consideration of a two-person interaction to the scenario of a multi-person interaction. A person lives in a community constituted by a number of others that are similar to him. He engages in a shared-semantic life embedded in this community. The awareness of others similar to himself, and with whom he can agree on some experiences, constitutes the basis for a communal semantic world. Aspects of experience shared by all individuals in the groups constitute the shared semantic life (culture) of the group (see Figure 5.4). Shared representations in a group serve as membership codes and protect the group from cheaters (see section 2.4).

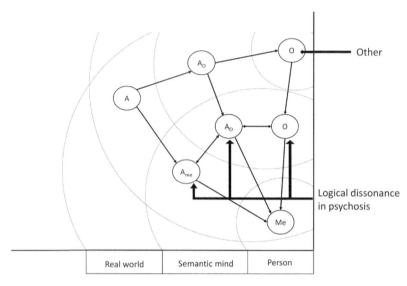

Figure 5.3. Representation of reality in psychosis. 'Me' is an experiencing agent that is experiencing psychosis. Ame is the representation of the world by 'me', distorted by psychopathology. Ao is other's representation of the world A. O represents others. When Ame and Ao are compared there is a dissonance that needs to be resolved, that is, why my experience of the world is different from others' experience of the same world. The discrepancy between Ame and Ao leads to logical dissonance in psychosis (see section 5.2.4).

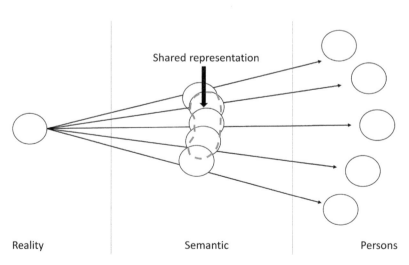

Figure 5.4. Representation of a group. Left: 'reality' in the empirical external world. Middle: shared representation of the empirical world by a group of individuals. Sharing is based on shared (overlapping) semantic representations enabled by language systems. Right: individual mental representations in different persons (see section 5.3).

5.3.1 Individual openness to group interaction

In development, an individual can exercise free choice in directing himself along a chosen development path. In a group context, he could choose the areas in which he wishes to be open to the influence of the group. Conversely, depending on the group, he may also wish to deliberately keep himself from some aspects of the shared group experiences (see Figure 5.5). For example, some people may choose to be less engaged with popular cultures in their community. A person choosing to be relatively closed to communal information may be open to other information. This information may be from another group (e.g., a member of a society or an online group), it can be semantic, that is, from books, or it can even be from the past (through books and through interaction with antiquities). If an individual is relatively distant to a group, he will not be able to update his social situation. Creative influence from a group may play a crucial role in individual development. Conversely, unhealthy influence from a group can compromise individual development. By active choice, the individual decides on a path of interaction that subsequently defines himself. In this manner the person can be considered as a product of the creative work of the person himself.

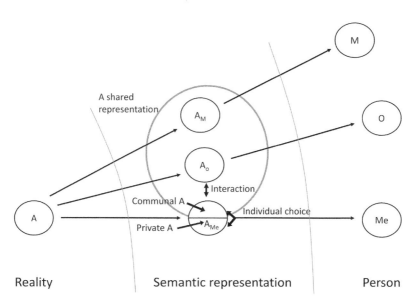

Figure 5.5. The role of individual choice in participation in the shared semantic world. A person exercises free choice in determining which of his mental representations engages with shared communal representations through interactions with others based on those mental representations. Such interactions increase the communal components and reduce the private components of the mental representations (see section 5.3.1).

6

Mental Representations as Containers for Information in Subjective Experiences

6.1 Development of Mental Representations

From birth, the brain embarks upon a one-way journey of plastic changes in relation to life experiences. The capacity of the brain to accommodate layers of information laid down progressively with time is a fundamental feature of human experience. Previous chapters have argued that it is possible to examine the structure of subjective experiences through phenomenology and to communicate them through an empathic dialogue process.

Subjective phenomena (experience) can be considered as being constructed from 'mental representations'. The contents of mental representations can be shared between two individuals using conversational dialogue. Even though the full personal meaning of the content of an experience may not be entirely exhaustible empirically, the use of dialogue can enable shareable information of an experience to be communicated. There are a number of ways through which mental representations have been explored in cognitive neuroscience. The 'parallel distributed processing' paradigm using constraint satisfaction is a simple but parsimonious model applicable to a wide range of representations. We propose to use this as a pragmatic tool to enable subjective experience to be handled as mental representations.

The development of mental representations emerges as the brain undergoes maturation in successive waves of critical periods during development (Rovee-Collier, 1995). Early acquisition determines basic cognitive structures such as the phoneme and lexical items during the early critical periods (Cheour et al., 1998). These basic cognitive structures may become the building blocks later for more complex structures (such as syntax and social schema) (DeWitt & Rauschecker, 2012). These structures are progressively built up in an orderly sequence of maturations in different brain systems. Critical periods are time windows during which the brain system is opened to environmental influences leading to active moulding of specific brain pathways (Slabakova, 2006). Different cognitive systems have specific critical periods (Eubank & Gregg, 1999). The maturation of different cognitive domains appears to follow a specifically timed sequence (Steinberg, 2005). During the critical period, the brain interacts with the environment to capture the regularities in the environment. The resulting connectivity becomes consolidated before the critical period time window is closed. Once the specific stage is passed, the brain moves on to the critical period for another domain. By adolescence the basic perceptual representations (such as the phoneme) are largely laid down. More complex representations may have a later time window; for example, the closure of the critical period time window for syntax representations may be around 17 years (Hartshorne et al., 2018; Lenneberg, 1967). Some authors have argued that faculties such as semantics may not have a closure time window (Slabakova, 2006).

Synaptic modification (e.g., pruning) in the prefrontal cortex takes place in late adolescence to enable long-term stability in higher order representations (e.g., social behaviour algorithms) to be established (Crews et al., 2007). In adult life, further changes become incremental and do not involve large-scale re-organization of brain connections. In youth, the brain undergoes transition from a childhood state of high pluripotency (ability to develop into a number of different possibilities) but lower efficiency to an adult state of high efficiency but lower pluripotency (Chechik et al., 1998; Craik & Bialystok, 2006; Hiratani & Fukai, 2015).

The adult brain is like a large organization consisting of many specialized teams. The team structure is allowed to evolve from an initially small amorphous group (i.e., in the child's brain) with 'every member communicating with everyone else and being involved in every task'. After the re-organization, more specialized roles emerge, with fewer connections between units. Further change is not in the basic structure but in the refinement of details.

Mental representations are 'information containers'. They receive, store, and update information. Importantly, they also act as templates for further information acquisition. Representations interact with the environment in a number of ways and time scales (see section 2.5). Low-level representation mediates moment-to-moment interaction with the perceptual information. Complex high-level representation mediates state of affairs (SOA) in the environment (situational models) and is revised continuously based on ongoing social information (see section 2.5.2). Also, the structure of high-level representations becomes enriched throughout personal development.

In early childhood, basic representations are initially formed by simple associations (corresponding to the Piagetian sensorimotor learning, Piaget & Inhelder, 1969). Subsequently, more comprehensive object representations are developed for the inanimate world (Piagetian object permanence, Piaget & Inhelder, 1969). This is followed by the development of mental representations of other people, using 'theories of mind' of increasing complexity (Astington & Jenkins, 1995). A theory of mind (TOM) is constructed based on interaction with others.

6.2 Representations in a Coherent Experience

Representations are structured clusters of information. Complex representations allow multi-faceted aspects of the environment to be depicted to enable more adaptive responses. We shall consider one example from animal behaviour.

Let us take the example of 'schooling': a fish swimming in a school of fishes while keeping its relative position constant in relation to other fishes. In schooling, the fish swims in a precise synchrony in the midst of a school of fishes, even amidst changing water currents (Pavlov & Kasumyan, 2000). We may consider in this case that the environment targets (position of the fish relative to other fishes) are internally computed as a relatively distinct unit (Hemelrijk & Hildenbrandt, 2012). In the human mind, when these distinct and co-occurring units of computation become part of the conscious experience, they constitute mental representations. Such unnamed 'sub-symbolic' fragments may be used and re-used in processing steps (MacDonald & MacDonald, 1995). Some would propose that these computations are used by the fish's perceptual and action systems in such a way that the fish is able to integrate itself into a larger system (the school of fishes) perfectly. Under such circumstances it is more profitable to consider the fish in the context of a larger system rather than the input and output in individual fishes. The more parsimonious view is to consider the entire school of fish as one single system. The connection between each component (individual fish) in the system is facilitated by the mirror neuron system, enabling very close synchrony between individual units. This perspective, when related to human experience, is echoed by Merleau-Ponty from a phenomenological perspective of Gestalt psychology: the Gestalt is 'a spontaneous organization of the sensory field' in which there are 'only organizations, more or less stable, more or less articulated' (Merleau-Ponty, 1933/1992).

The schooling example engages an action-perception (AP) mental representation that is relatively simple. It is likely that complex representations are developed in humans to engage the social environment (Zwaan & Radvansky, 1998). This involves probabilistic computation for high-dimensional 'mental states', enabling game-theoretic consideration of others (conspecifics with game-playing strategies) as active agents (capable of making choices) (O'Brien et al., 1998).

Complex representations (consisting of an organized group of simple representations) are constructed as 'argument-predicate' propositional structures to indicate possible SOAs in the environment (Hurford, 2003). An example SOA representation is: 'I think Peter has received a present from Mary.' In this example, the mental representations for Peter, Mary, the present, and the act of receiving a present are constructed to represent a social scenario. It is important to note that the representation can be set up regardless of whether it is a true reflection of the real world. The person 'I' relates to this representation in a somewhat tentative reflective manner (the 'I think' component). The fact that they are modular units allow them to be handled flexibly as components open to re-combination in creative processes (Pinker, 1994). They can represent states

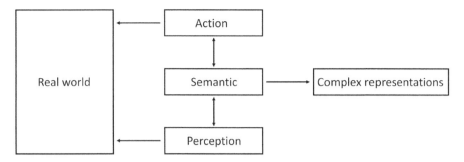

Figure 6.1. The content of subjective experiences may involve action, semantic, and perceptual representations (see section 6.1). Action and perception representations are relatively bound to the empirical external world. Semantic (complex) representations are more open to manipulation in the mind. The links between action, perception and semantic mental representations enable flexible and manoeuvrable mental representations.

in reality or in imagination (see section 3.4.1). States can be located in the future or in the past. Representations can be assigned information value according to a process discussed previously (see section 2.5 on information).

The types of mental representations involved in the content of subjective experiences can be perceptual (touch, taste, smell), action (initiating a well-learnt movement), or semantic (words and propositions, including symbolic imagery and visualization). Actions are only expressed in the present moment. Perceptual representations are stimulus-bound in the present moment and less subjected to internal manipulations. They are thus 'primordial' (see section 5.2). Mental representations in the perceptual and action streams are connected and shared and can be used interchangeably (the AP model, Prinz, 1997). Semantic representations, on the other hand, are less stimulus-bound and are more open to mental manipulations. Mapping between semantic, perceptual, and action representations (concepts) allows perceptual and action representations to be used in rich combinations (see Figure 6.1). Through the connection to semantic units, action and perceptual representations can be freed from stimulus bondage and handled more flexibly in the mind through the links to semantic representation. However, when a predominantly 'semantic' mode of operation (thinking mode) is involved, the representations are less filled with perceptual details compared with the 'perceptual' mode (see section 3.5.1).

The experience of the mind corresponds to the Lifeworld in phenomenology. The Lifeworld can be communicated through language in a shared semantic net (see section 1.4 on language and subjectivity). This semantic world can be accessed through interpersonal dialogues (see section 1.4.1 on ethnography).

Importantly, mental representations are not static entities. They are instantiated at the moment of activation (Rumelhart et al., 1987a). Upon activation, a network of nodes is also invoked. These co-activations contribute to accessing the meaning associated with the representations.

In handling incoming information, the brain parses out 'background or contextual' information from 'foreground' information (Goldstein, 1939). De-contextualization of episodic representations necessitates the existence of a 'difference-same' comparison in the brain, parsing the input into more invariant fragments (background context) as well as more specific (foreground) information. This basic operation generates modular units of information representing relatively stable and discrete elements in the environment (see section 2.5).

6.2.1 States of Affairs are represented as propositions

An SOA is a complex mental representation about the state of the external world (Zwaan & Radvansky, 1998). SOAs are constructed from simple representations of objects and actions organized in a structured manner. They often follow the structure of propositional statements in language (e.g., A sees B hitting C) (see Figure 6.2, SOA of language). They are expected to have a truth value (i.e., they can be considered as true or false). Even false SOA representations are valid representations in the mind and are important for mental activities (e.g., in imagination or in counterfactual thinking).

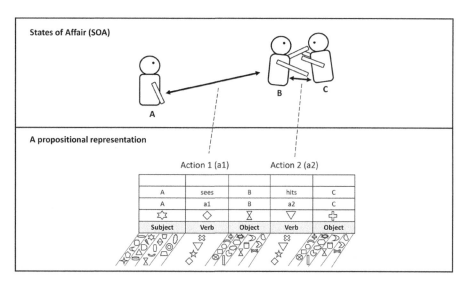

Figure 6.2. States of Affairs (SOAs) are formulated as propositions. Actions are involved in the SOAs. These states are expressed in a propositional statement in the human mind (see section 6.2.1). In this example A sees (action) B hit (action) C. 'B hit C' is an SOA embedded in A sees [B hit C]. Such embedding is enabled by the propositional structure of mental representations.

6.2.2 Mutuality in a network of representations

In the process of knowing, we build an understanding of the world with concepts (mental representations) (see Figure 6.3). This process of building up is continuous. The self 're-positions' itself continuously in relation to the represented world in an adaptive manner. In this process, the 'meanings' of individual objects are *constructed*. The representations of objects thus generated are linked to one another and mutually relate to one another by providing two-way contributions to meanings (Deacon, 1997). *One representation makes full sense only in relation to other representations* and vice versa. This cross-support between representations also introduces the possibilities of creating *novel meanings*. Novel meanings can be found in new objects not yet encountered and may not map to a 'real' external object (e.g., they can map to mythical objects).

6.3 Mental Representations of Objects

Mental representations (mental models, concepts, or ideas) mediate how the mind relates to objects in the world (see section 2.3). They also help the human mind to place objects within a coherent system of meaning (Kempson, 1988). Representations can be simple, mapping directly to an external object. They can also be complex, in the form of a situational model with propositional structure, referring to an SOA in the external world (see section 2.3). Here we elaborate more on the different classes of objects that are represented.

A semantic network

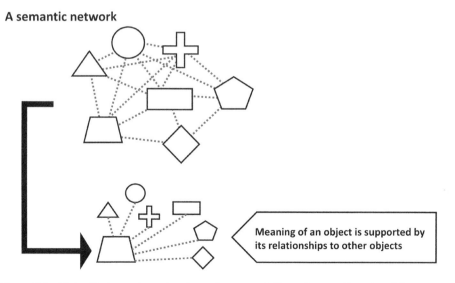

Meaning of an object is supported by its relationships to other objects

Figure 6.3. Mutuality in a coherent system of representations. A semantic network is represented by a cluster of interconnected concepts (shapes). In a semantic network, the meaning of an object is partially derived from its links to other objects (see section 6.2.2).

6.3.1 Categories of represented objects: Things, material substance, and forms

Propositions with a structure 'A is B' are often used to communicate information about the 'what' in our world (Zwaan & Radvansky, 1998). The 'information value' of a proposition 'A is B' depends on how common 'B' is. This determines how redundant the proposition 'A is B' is. From an information perspective, if B is common, the statement contains less information, and if B is rare, the statement contains more information.

6.3.2 'Things' as 'material objects' and 'ideas' as non-material 'forms'

We consider how material and form interact using the example of a teapot. When we relate to a particular teapot in daily use, we are treating it as a specific *material object* in our mind. However, a potter making a teapot starts with clay as the material and imparts the 'form' of a teapot to the clay material. The 'form' partly consists of the generic 'idea' of the teapot and partly of what characterizes this present individual teapot. The form is considered as something beyond material matter. It contains information. Through their forms, created 'artefacts' are meaningful to human beings (Stein, 1931/1998). In our example, this corresponds to the generic concept of a teapot.

6.3.3 Information in forms

As opposed to matter, the 'form' is a salient informational structure engaging the human mind. In material things, it is often the 'form' that is related to the function of the object, as opposed to the material from which it is made (Aristoteliam *Materie*, scholastic *prima materia*, Aristotle, 1999). Forms are patterns of correlated features. They can be shaped by a creative input (with the imparting of information) giving forms to matter. Mankind can create forms by shaping, but mankind cannot create matter (Andrieu, 2006).

'Forms' concern us more than 'matter' in daily life. When we wish to make tea, we first think of the idea of a teapot (an idea in the informational realm) rather than the clay that makes up the teapot (in the physical substance realm). The form of the teapot consists of its components, the spout, the body, the handle, the foot, and the cover. Each of these components can take up a specific option amongst a range of options (e.g., the spout can be long or short, the body can be rounded or squared, the foot can be high or low). The selection of each option involves information. There are also constraints between the different parts: a round body is usually associated with a round cover, a large handle is usually related to a long spout, and the spout cannot be lower than the height of the body. The information contained in the teapot thus consists of the various options in the specific components (e.g., low foot, small handle). Information is also contained in the correlations (constraints) between patterns; for example, rounded cover is associated with rounded body. This correlation is also informational in that given feature A (the shape of the cover) the possible options for feature B will be narrowed down (the shape of body).

6.3.4 Forms and cognitive representations

Forms can be 'filled' by specific instances (individual exemplars), as a biological species (a form) is filled by the actual individuals. There are features in empty forms that are filled differently by different individual exemplars. Forms can be considered as a feature template that has several dimensions. These dimensions can be filled with different possibilities (Hinton, 1989).

In the example of the teapot, the idea of teapot is a 'form' in contrast to an actual particular teapot (that small pear-shaped red-clay Yi-xiang teapot I bought two years ago).

In the representation of a teapot (see Figure 6.4), there are features that correspond to a generic teapot (e.g., shape, size, handle). The feature space is laid out but does not need to be filled, except for the defining features of a teapot (e.g., has a spout, can contain water), which need to be filled in the affirmative. A representation with feature space outlined but unfilled corresponds to a *conceptual* type of representation. Filling in *specific* contents in the feature space will render a *perceptual* type of representation

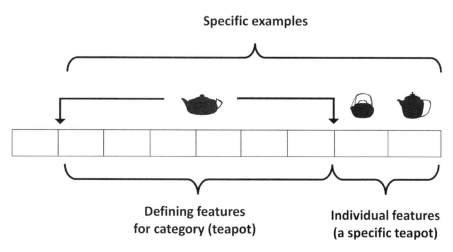

Specific examples

**Defining features
for category (teapot)**

**Individual features
(a specific teapot)**

Figure 6.4. Category representations and 'forms'. Using 'teapots' as an example of a category or a 'form' that exists in the information world. The information contained in the form of teapots consists of core dimensions of a teapot (e.g., the shape, the function, the parts such as the cover, the handle, the spout); then there are optional features (such as the material, the size, the proportion the foot), When the 'Form' of a teapot category is used to represent a specific teapot, the defining features are first endorsed and then the unique feature dimensions are 'filled' by specification of these dimensions for the individual teapot, for example, a clay teapot with a long curved spout (see section 6.3.5).

of a particular teapot (e.g., tall, small, metal; see section 2.3). For the individual teapot, there may also be additional feature dimensions beyond that of a general teapot (e.g., the actual shape, the special use).

In the Japanese tea ceremony (Sencha do), different utensils are specified to be used in different stages. The 'form' specifies a particular utensil type (e.g., a summer tea caddy). However, the individual utensil (such as the teapot) is selected from a pool of possible teapots on a specific occasion, depending on the particular theme for the particular ceremony, the season, and the guests. This selection of individual utensils is purposeful and informational; thus it can be considered as a creative action. The tea ceremony itself lays out a complex mega-representation specifying the utensils needed for each part of the ceremony. The teapot is one of the utensils. The generic teapot representation is embedded in the mega-representation of the tea ceremony. When the ceremony is actualized on a specific occasion, the use of a particular teapot fills out the representation and conveys information and meaning to the participants.

6.3.5 Nuance of experience activated by intersecting layers in the semantic net

Husserl (1890–1908/1993) recognized an important issue in the subjective experience of categories. In experiencing an object with red colour, there is *at the same time* perceptions of the 'specific redness' and the 'generic redness'. Both the specific and the generic are experienced *at the same time*. A full experience is one where both specific and general experiences are simultaneously received.

Ancient Chinese philosopher Kung-sun Long has highlighted this issue in his famous 'white horse' problem posed around 300 BC (Fung, 1958). Kung-sun argued that 'a white horse is not a horse'. He explained the term 'horse' is colour-neutral, and it therefore differs from 'white horse'. Based on these two different terms, when 'horse' is used, one points to horses regardless of colour. However, when 'white horse' is used, any creature not white will not be regarded as the object. The logical problem concerns a mismatch in the layers of the semantic universe in which the problem was framed. What is poignant for us is the realization that when we see a white horse, we simultaneously experience a 'white horse' as well as a 'horse'. Indeed, we also have experience of 'whiteness' associated with the 'white horse'. Thus the experience represents an intersection of representations with the 'horseness' and 'whiteness', as well as this particular white horse in front of us (see Figure 6.5).

In experiencing, we perceive a particular object from the specific attributes of that object. At the same time some general attributes, for example, whiteness, and the concepts constituting those attributes (whiteness) are activated and experienced (see Figure 6.5). These general concepts can also become objects of mental acts. When someone sees a white horse, a generic horse is also experienced. They are respectively experienced as the 'particular' and the 'general' (Husserl, 1913, 1921/1970).

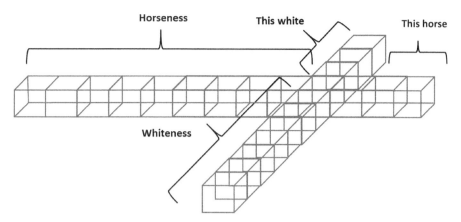

Figure 6.5. Representation for 'this white horse' activates the generic representations of 'whiteness' and 'horseness'. In perceiving a white horse, there is at the same time activation of the more general representations for 'horseness' and for 'whiteness' (see section 6.3.6). The simultaneous co-activation of special representation and more generic representation is an important feature giving rise to multi-layer quality of subjective experience.

The 'general' representation is co-located with the 'particular' but is separable. In the semantic network, activating one exemplar will activate the different conceptual layers to shape a particular semantic environment, and in perceiving one object, one attribute will activate the whole conceptual framework (e.g., this white horse, white horses, horses, whiteness, animals, colours, and living things). The activation of such a layered hierarchy of representations allows for the subtle nuance in daily subjective experiences. These considerations are important for psychopathology as often the representations may not be complete in all feature dimensions. Information about which dimensions are filled and which are not filled is important in psychopathology.

In daily life, the relative activation of the different layers of features in a representation depends on the context in which the concept is activated. When one is only concerned with making tea, the core teapot representation is activated and dominates (e.g., material becomes secondary, and whether it is a metal or ceramic teapot matters less). When one is considering making tea for a number of people, then the size dimension becomes relatively important. If the tea-making is for a group of friends who enjoy teawares, then the material and the shape, and indeed the cultural context, of the teapot may be relatively important. The relative activation of the various feature dimensions has to be flexibly adapted to the occasion. This process of flexibly and adaptively setting up the representational space according to the context is computationally intensive and may be compromised. For instance, when a fast decision is required, the number of features that is considered may be reduced, resulting in excessive weight being assigned to a small number of features. Stereotypes, heuristics, biases can often arise in these situations. In disorders that affect executive functions, inadequate resources for setting up of an adaptive representation may compromise judgement and social functions, resulting in behaviour and cognitions that may be considered as inflexible. In times of group conflicts, polarizing in-group and out-group phenomena often label people as 'them' and 'us' and reduce the individual person to a member of a category (the phenomena of dehumanization). Extensive digital communication may intensify reduction of representational dimensions, as short text messages and rapid response time often limit the setting up of full feature spaces for representations. When categorization is based on limited information, biased conclusions may arise (jumping to conclusions). The initial inaccurate conclusions may prime (provide context for) the setting up of subsequent feature space so that information inconsistent with the initial impression is more difficult to be considered subsequently (Bias Against Disconfirmatory Evidence). These behaviours have been observed in people with tendencies towards psychotic disorders, suggesting that inadequate setting up of representational space might be an important contributor towards psychotic experiences.

6.3.6 Forms in the mind

Forms are important as they represent the non-material and informational aspects of experience. Pure forms are distinct from matter (emptied of contents). They *exist by themselves* in the *realms of the 'spirit'* (*Geistwesen*, Hegel, 1807/1977). They are ideas and concepts (e.g., whiteness) that have a life of their own in their own realms of existence. This realm of ideas is also the realm for human creative action. For example, the creative mind may design a teapot in the shape of a fruit, for the use with fruit teas. A highly creative designer may even conceive a new type of utensil beyond existing types or forms. When this happens, a new conceptual space is created for the new 'utensil' (e.g., some large shiny cylindrical mugs in the Renaissance period might possibly be used for deciphering secretly coded images through its concave reflection, this then developing into the art form of anamorphic cylindrical images).

6.3.7 Mutuality amongst symbols: Hidden semantic corners

In the semantic net, some concepts (symbols) point to external objects. Direct experience with the external objects (as referents) gives primary meaning to the symbol. When a number of related concepts are linked to one another and weaved into a network (see Figure 6.6), each can derive some of their meanings from cross-referencing between concepts. A collection of concepts thus derives meaning from one another in a mutually supportive network (e.g., the concepts of doctor, nurse, patients, hospitals, and illness support each other) (Deacon, 1997; Solé et al., 2010).

It is important to emphasize that given a particular population of interacting words with their individual meanings, some new possibilities for meaning are already poignant before a new word is actually constructed to express them (Wisniewski, 1997).

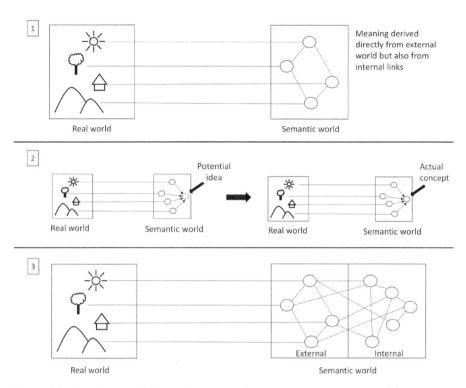

Figure 6.6. Development of internally generated representations. 1: regions of the semantic net that directly encode aspects of the external world. 2: new 'internal' nodes that can be formed solely by relationship with other semantic nodes. These internal nodes do not have direct mapping to the external world. 3: interconnections between the network of internal nodes, as well as the real-world regularities constraints internal nodes (see section 6.3.6).

There is thus a 'top-down' aspect to semantic nets. Meaning can be generated internally apart from external references.

For example, the idea of an 'airport' may have existed before the first airport was built. The idea was made poignant with the progress in air travel. The idea of 'air travel' blended with the idea of 'ports' (initially that of a seaport) to produce the idea of an airport. The meaning of the airport was already 'in existence' in the inner semantic net of people even before a word was used to express the idea. In this case, we can use the regularity of our semantic net to project into the future; should space travel be commercializable, there will be 'space-ports'. If one uses this term, most people will probably get the meaning even though the word might not have been in existence. Ideas can be conceivable in the collective mind even when actual objects are not (yet) encountered in real life.

In the human mind some 'potentials' for meaning are also commonly expressed in folklore. Anthropologists have studied the shared structures and themes amongst folktales of different cultures. These meanings are internally formed and do not require explicit external referent. Some psychopathological experiences (e.g., neologism) may also be linked with these 'inner semantic corners' (Fauconnier & Turner, 2008).

6.3.8 Parsing and co-segregating of semantic fragments

It is proposed that the brain, upon receiving information from the environment, identifies sets of repeatedly encountered co-occurring regularities. It extracts and groups them into co-segregating clusters. This parsing of incoming information is required as a back-engineering process to fractionate a complex episodic representation into a number of separable representations (see Figure 6.2), as in the process of perception. This process is important in identifying regularities in the environment (see Figure 6.6) (Stickgold, 2005; Wiedemann, 2007). The grouping of co-occurring information is the foundation for the identification of discrete units of representations. From a mechanistic point of view, there is no reason that the parsing should respect boundaries set by our conscious mind. The fragments may not correspond to 'nameable' conceptual constructs, ideas, or emotions. Representations at these levels have been described as 'sub-symbolic' (Smolensky, 1995).

When we perceive sounds from the environment, our auditory system engages in an 'auditory scene analysis' (Bregman, 1990). It parses the composite auditory input into different 'streams'. For example, the air conditioner background noise is placed into one stream, the occasional hammering noise from the next building into another stream, the speech noise from 'A' talking to me into yet another stream. The verbal sounds of 'A' are further parsed into the basic voice (of 'A', invariant) and the phonemes (changes rapidly, maps to meaning). The initial sound waves arriving at my ears are composite vibrations involving all these overlapping streams. The auditory system 'reverse engineers' and unpacks the component streams, most of the time successfully. The more constant (background) components become the template (structure) that interacts with the more variable, individualized foreground components to identify a specific individual.

6.3.9 Offline consolidation of information

Human memory does not transit straight from registration to storage. An intermediate state is required in which the hippocampus plays essential functions before the memory trace is deposited elsewhere in the cortex for long-term storage (Miller, 1991; Rolls, 1989; Squire, 1987). It has been suggested that one of the functions during this period of consolidation is to allow for a tentative holding of memory traces 'in buffer' where they are allowed to interact with existing memory, as well as further incoming memories, in order to arrive at a representation more coherent with other representations before being committed to long-term storage (Bliss & Lomo, 1973; Malenka & Bear, 2004).

During the wakeful alert state, representations are continuously 'engaged' with external perception. Consolidation of information appears to require sleep and dreaming and cannot take place effectively in the wakeful state (Paller & Voss, 2004; Wamsley, 2014) (see Figure 6.7).

Our daily experiences are constructed from representations that have a semantic component as well as a perceptual component. It is interesting to note that in dreams, the experience is mainly perceptual rather than semantic. Studies of dream reports suggest that dreams often have visual components and less often have verbal components. One interpretation of the free-flowing visual perceptual content of dreams is that they may represent the 'tail-ends' of representations that are freely available to the dream contents' awareness platform. The core process of consolidation may engage the other parts of the representations, that is, the verbal, context-bound components at the other 'front ends' of the representations (the verbal semantic links) (Buckner et al., 2008; Paller & Voss, 2004; Stickgold, 1998; Wamsley & Stickgold, 2010).

6.4 Domains of Experiences Represented

To consider the potentials of using 'representations' to address subjective experience, some important domains of representations in the human mind are considered here (see Figure 6.8). It is important to recall that a fundamental feature of the mind is to relate (see section 3.5 on relating). These domains are where the objects for 'relating' are located. In a psychopathological investigation, one of the primary objectives is to access and clarify representations.

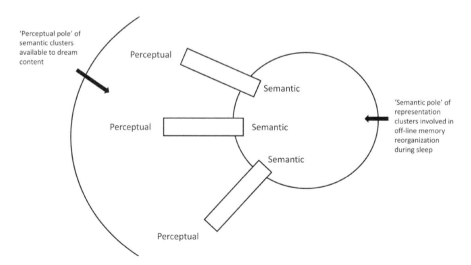

Figure 6.7. Semantic and perceptual information in sleep. During offline re-organization of semantic contents in memory during REM sleep, the associated perceptual information may be made available to dream contents (see section 6.3.9).

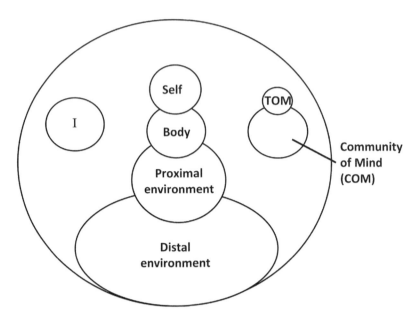

Figure 6.8. Important content domains of representations in the human mind. Distal environment overlaps with proximal environment, body, and self; COM consists of TOMs of a group of individuals (see section 6.3).

6.4.1 Representation of the self

Self-representation is involved in the basic momentary phenomena of '*cogito sum*', as a transitory but experiencing, relating, and acting awareness (see section 3.2.1 on being). There is also the 'third-person' awareness of the self, as one of the many similar individuals in existence and as being located in the external world. Awareness of the self develops in the second year of life before the emergence of language. The sense of self appears to have developed through the processes of joint attention (Tomasello & Call, 1997). Infants initially explore the world through sensory motor engagement. They learn about the world through active exploration in the first person. The infant learns about the mother and relates to her. Then a uniquely human process takes place. The infant learns to refer to (point to) a third object in the environment and engages the mother's attention towards that object (joint attention). The next development is that the infant learns that they themselves are the object of attention. This opens the possibility of the infant considering themselves from a third-person perspective. Eventually the first-person experience and third-person views become integrated and an initial but comprehensive self-awareness emerges. The experience of agency (awareness of action initiation by self) is vital to self-representation (David et al., 2008; Gallagher, 2000; Haggard et al., 2002; Hohwy, 2007; Northoff et al., 2006; Synofzik et al., 2009).

Representations of 'others' in relation to the self is an important consideration (Schneider et al., 2008). Objects have varying degrees of proximity to the self. Others that are closely related to the self could be relatively more influenced by active control through agency and represent the part of the world that is relatively controllable by the self (see section 6.1 on developing person). However, others are never completely predictable or controllable. Disturbances in self-relatedness attributes are involved in psychotic experiences (van Buuren et al., 2012).

After the emergence of a third-person perspective, the relationship between the self and others can be represented as propositions just like the relationship between two external others. The representation involves 'the self', a relationship/action, and 'the other'. Such a relationship contributes to the characterization of the self. Often a reciprocal relationship exists between the self and the others (when I perceive another person as strong, I am perceiving myself as weak in relation to that person).

6.4.2 Representation of the body

Body representation involves the body schema, such as the spatial representation of the body (mediated by the non-dominant parietal cortex). First-person experiences of the body are accomplished through direct sensory feedback of movement from joint positions, visceral sensations, touch, and so forth (Damasio, 1996; Vogeley & Fink, 2003). Visual exploration of oneself through a mirror is a special case (Gallup et al., 2014; Mitchell, 1993; Schwenkler, 2008). Experiencing action through the sense of agency is also an important part of self-experience (Martin, 1995). The impact of body representation on general cognition (embodiment) is increasingly being recognized (Carruthers, 2007; Eilan et al., 1995). For example, it is easier to concentrate better whilst sitting down compared with standing up or during exercise. Cognitive linguistics highlighted the role of body representation in the construction of basic semantic concepts (Carruthers, 2007; Damasio, 1994). It is increasingly recognized that body representation is basic to experiencing the material world. Body presentation generates basic models of experiencing through which more abstract experience can be constructed (Johnson & Lakoff, 2002; Lakoff, 2012).

Spatial experience of the self has also been explored in phenomenology (e.g., zero point of reference, see sections 4.4 and 4.5; Stein, 1916/1970). Spatial reference is one of the starting points of empathy towards other people. Body experience is thus important in empathy and the representation of others. For example, through the mirror neuron system (Rizzolatti et al., 1996), bodily self-experience can be linked with that of other individuals, creating a possibility of connecting the representations of inner states of sensation between the self and others (Gallese & Goldman, 1998; Gallese et al., 2004). The mirror neurons in the prefrontal cortex are activated when the subject observes an intentional movement in another individual. This results in subthreshold activation in the observer's mirror neurons corresponding to the observed action. For example, when the observer sees another person move a hand to pick up a cup, the mirror neurons in the observer corresponding to the same hand movement are activated in the observer's prefrontal cortex. When an observer observes facial expression suggestive of pain, mirror neurons associated to pain expression muscles are activated in the observer, resulting in a partial activation of the same facial expression in the observer. This action facilitates the retrieval of a sensation of pain in the observer. The mirror neuron provides a brain account for empathy in non-verbal communications.

Disturbance of body representation is involved in a number of mental conditions. In anorexia nervosa there is a distortion in body image. In dysmorphophobia there is also a delusional distortion in self appearance. Delusion of offensive smell arising from oneself is a common experience in psychosis.

6.4.3   Representation of the proximal environment

The proximal environment represents the part of the environment that is in close proximity to the individual, for instance, personal space, home, and accessories. Importantly it is defined not only by physical proximity but also by 'informational proximity'. From the 'information' perspective, the proximal environment is one in which the person has relatively good mastery and control. It is a 'realm' where the individual can largely predict. It is often a familiar environment associated with a sense of security. The proximal environment is not restricted to physical space. Cyberspace may play an increasingly important role.

The environment that a person inhabits and manages is a space in which personalized preferences are actualized. The person chooses to engage in some options over others. The environment can be differentiated into more controllable and less controllable domains. In daily life much energy is invested into shaping this proximal environment by personal choices. This cumulates to give a sense of personal identity. The act of choosing produces organized information that eventually conveys a sense of identity for the individual.

A special compartment in the proximal environment is the set of personal accessories. This includes objects that are carried in close physical proximity by the individual most of the time. Their presence evokes a sense of security. They can also be displayed to express individual identity. Personal accessories are particularly poignant with meaning and information. The material nature of accessories matters far less (see section 4.2.2). Their 'personalization' has long been recognized and respected. The ancient practice of burial objects is a manifestation of the close relationship between humans and personal objects.

A particularly poignant example is found in the traditional 'study' of oriental scholars in the past. The study is a proximal environment for the intellectual. However, it need not be material. Indeed, there are many studies that are mostly virtual, existing only in the mind and poems of the impoverished scholar (i.e., informational). In the modern era, the digital world provides an important personalized proximal environment. The proximal environment is safe, but as a rule, people may also prefer some elements of unpredictability. The proximal environment thus constitutes a base from which more adventurous exploration can take place in the distal environment. Hoarding and collecting in the proximal environment reflect a specific mode of relating between the individual and his proximal world.

6.4.4 Representation of the distal environment

The distal environment consists of the 'external world at large'. In this environment there are 'knowns' and 'unknowns'. Many events are beyond personal knowledge and control. The environment is rich, is varied, and has a broad spatial and temporal span. The distal environment has physical and geographical dimensions, but it also has social, semantic, and informational dimensions (e.g., in the library of Babel or the online world) (Borges, 1941/1962; Leiner et al., 1997). The distal environment gives us a perspective that we exist as transitory beings in a more extensive and longer lasting world that each of us individually cannot totally exhaust. Aspects of the distal environment become internalized in the proximal environment in the process of our learning and integration of new experiences. An instinctive appetite for information drives this process of exploration in the new environment and in the mastery of new space and new skills. It also drives mankind in the mastery of knowledge. Consummation of information, driven by curiosity, is a basic mode in which humans relate to their world. Human experiences are also founded upon a pragmatic sense that we share the distal environment with other individuals.

6.4.5 Representation of the extended empirical world

The empirical world can also be explored by instruments that extend the range of human experience (such as the telescope and the microscope). Through such instruments we expand our sensory range. Through scientific notations and concepts, we grasp laws of nature and re-constitute a perspective of our world that is richer and enables more powerful predictions. It is however important to realize the limitations of this empirical mode of experiencing the world. Because of its overwhelming richness, it is easy for individuals to be lost while trying to engage in this seemingly inexhaustible world. This leads to an impoverished position that the empirical world is the only reality that one can engage with. It is important to appreciate that the empirical world, rich as it is, constitutes only a portion of 'experienceable' possibilities in human life.

6.4.6 Representation of others

The representation of other individuals in the world gives rise to a shared objectivity that is the foundation for knowing the external world (see Chapter 5 on empathy; Stein, 1916/1970). The consideration of other individuals as equivalent to ourselves is a fundamental position in the human condition. It necessitates the use of 'semi-autonomous representations' to approximate the complexity in others (Lewis, 2002). The use of semi-autonomous representations was first explicitly used by novel writers, who wrote not according to a predetermined plot but allowed the characters in the novel, each with their individuality, to 'freely' interact and determine the outcome of the story. In this way the writer has to be open to developments that might surprise even himself. This open attitude enables the treatment of other individuals as similar to ourselves. The position of treating others as less than ourselves has been described as 'existential inauthenticity' (Buber, 1925/1937; Macquarrie, 1972). This position is related to 'dehumanization' and its related negative consequences (Haslam, 2006).

6.4.7 Representation of groups

Representation of the social group in which we are situated consists of not only the individual representations of others but also of the representations of the relationship between individuals. This includes those to whom one might not have direct access. Inferences and deductions are used to compute these indirect hidden links. Semi-autonomous representations are deployed to represent members of the group. The group SOA is continuously monitored for new information. Representation of groups are costly and potentially limited by the brain cortical size (Dunbar, 1996). It is one of the important domains in which erroneous conclusions can emerge in mental conditions, for example, in giving rise to persecutory delusions and third-person hallucinations.

6.4.8 Representation of the Divine

Representation of the Divine is universal across human cultures. Different religious faiths attest to human aspirations to relate to the Divine. What emerged was an abstract concept of the Divine (the Creator) to which the limited human mind fails to properly relate. In the Divine representation, some feature dimensions are being filled at infinity values (power, knowledge, size and guarantor of human values, i.e., 'all-loving').

In relating to the Divine, the appropriate position to adopt may be that of a 'creaturely' position (Pryzwara, 2014; Stein, 1916/1970). One has to concede that human mental representations are likely to be inadequate. Human-initiated attempts to grasp the Divine have, not surprisingly, been met with limited success and resulted in the repeated cultural phenomena of human attempts to define and institutionalize religion (Geertz, 1973).

'Revelation' enables a new way of relating. Instead of the self relating as an active subject, humans can position themselves as recipients to receive aspects of Divine information that is actively revealed to sapiens (Barth, 1957/1961).

In the Christian faith, God introduced Christ as a participating human being. In terms of representations this is unique amongst religions. A 'person' representation is adopted to represent the Divine. The representation of a person has a different structure from the general, more abstract representation of other objects, as well as the representation of the Divine as a concept. This enables a unique possibility for human creatures to relate in a more tangible manner to the divine person. This relationship can potentially bring humans out of solitary entrapment in the biological and semantic levels of existence.

The roles that a divine representation plays in individual mental life can be pivotal. 'Divine representation' is all-knowing, thus all of one's thoughts are open to the divine. God is also conceived as omnipotent, thus the prime mover, which sets a context in which we understand our own agency as a given, a gift. We are free to choose only insofar as we are given this freedom by God through an act of withholding the overriding presence of Himself in the spheres of our existence (Yu, 1988). The positioning of the divine representation in relation to the 'self' reveals whether our self is too narrowly located in the centre of our representations.

Responding to the Divine humbles us and at the same time enables us to reach beyond the narrow human-centred perspective, just as responding to others enables us to emerge from narcissism. The risk of narcissism also depends on how we locate our own representations of the Divine. In modern culture the representation of God is often downplayed. The study of a person's divine representation or their lack thereof is important in the understanding of the person.

6.4.9   Representation in the digital world

In this section we shall consider the implications of increasing digitalization to human experiences. Recent decades have witnessed an acceleration in the taking up of digital technology in many facets of human experiences. Hardly any area of human activity is left untouched by digital 'innovations'. The internet and the mobile phone have brought the digital world into the proximal environment for many people. The time spent in interaction with the digital world occupies a significant proportion of the waking life. For most people the time spent in digital interaction is not a well-demarcated block of time but is distributed and inserted into different activities throughout the day. The engagement with digital activity on the smartphone is multi-faceted. Typically, the engagement is in small units, with only a short time spent on any unit before switching to another task. The activity often involves simple reception of a message, the selection of a response (such as an emoticon) from a range of possibilities, or the sending of truncated short text messages.

The increased share of the digital world in human experiences is driven by an important factor. In contrast to the material world, the digital world is less limited by resources. Objects in the material world are space-occupying and require a physical material substrate. Both space and material are finite resources. Once space and material are committed to one object, in general they cannot be available to other objects at the same time. For digital objects such limitation is much less severe. The implementation of digital objects is on a micro-scale in silicon chips and optic fibres. Once implemented they can be accessed by millions of people (e.g., a website). The digital object is an 'information object' that does not consume limited material and spatial resources. Once created, digital objects can be distributed to millions of people at little additional costs. There is thus a shift of the limit from the producer to the consumer (device, bandwidth, and the time and mental capacity of the human receiver). Moreover, removal of the material resource limitation renders the choice of digital experience potentially without bound. The individual therefore experiences an unprecedented range of choice in the digital world. Access to knowledge, utilities, entertainment, and social interaction has become readily available over the digital platform. The individual thereby experiences an unrivalled sense of control over his environment. While the contents of the digital environment (such as access to scenery of a distant location) corresponds to the distal environment, they can now be accessed with the ease and control that were previously available only in the proximal environment. Rapid increased engagement with the digital world is expected to increase the proportion of encounters that are experienced as being directly controllable by the subject. The sense of individual choice and agency appears to be unparalleled in the history of mankind.

Despite this apparent progress, there are some problems with the advent of digital technology. The experience of surprise and novelty in an encounter has become less common. Associated with this is the loss of a sense of uniqueness and personalization in human experience. Digital experience becomes 'cheap' in human transactions. Acquisition and sharing of experience are less costly and can be conducted *en masse*. The increased control and lack of surprise in the digital world imply that the digital experience is perceived as predictable in most digital domains. Given the innate drive to engage with exploration in the human mind (see section 3.5), those areas in the digital world that are less predictable will be selectively more engaging. These areas include social media, online shopping and auctions, gaming, gambling, and video experiences. They are indeed amongst the most popular activities in the digital world. In contrast, the informational, and instructional aspects of the digital world appear less engaging.

The multi-faceted use of the mobile phone (social media, weather, scheduling, photography, etc.) in daily life demands multiple switching between tasks. Switching is costly in terms of cognitive resources. Multiple switching between a large number of trivial but mildly reinforcing daily tasks (such as social media) can drain cognitive resources. When cognitive resources are depleted, self-control is reduced, resulting in more entrapment in simple, passive, non-creative, digital engagement and over-use of the digital media.

The easy access to a wide range of digital experience and the constant availability of choices mean that more difficult, more effortful experiences may be shunted off in preference for easier experiences. When more challenging engagement is required in an area, it is relatively easy for the subject to switch to a less challenging area. As a result, there will likely be selective engagement with relatively less effortful areas. Challenges to the comfort zone in order to engage the best within individual potentials will be more likely to be left unfulfilled and uncompleted (see section 4.1). This results in more shallow and more fragmented, but more relaxed, life experiences. The ready availability of the mobile phone enables the filling of time gaps that were previously left unoccupied. For example, moments in transit (e.g., in an elevator) and moments in a queue used to be unfilled time gaps that were often left for resting brain activities such as daydreaming and light reflection (see section 6.7). Access to the digital media has now replaced daydreaming and reflective experiences. This has resulted in a shift of experience to the external digital world from the inner world of the self. Less opportunity is available for the processing of information in the inner self-related domains. With digitalization there is thus a shift of experience from the private individual domain to the shareable external digital domain. The shareable external digital domain is also more shallow and less nuanced. The use of language is less complex in the digital world, with short text messages and emoticons replacing conventional language expressions. This may result in less nuanced modes or relating between the self and experiential life domains. The externalization of experience to shallow digital platforms (which become the new intersubjective platform) means that the semantic meaning structure can be more easily controlled by external agents who have control over contents and their associations.

Moreover, the widespread availability of the online platform has promoted the democratization of knowledge. Not only is knowledge widely accessible, the expression of judgement and opinion has become widespread in the online platform. In the previous material-based world, knowledge was a sought-after commodity institutionalized in, for example, universities. The public assigned knowledge-making roles to specialized professionals. Professional judgements and opinions were trusted by individuals. In the digital age, there is more involvement of the individual in coming into contact with knowledge and research. Many opinion leaders have emerged. They replace the traditional experts. Topics are treated with less depth and people form an opinion more easily, driven by popular online expressions and dissemination of information.

The effects of increased online engagement, increased information possibilities, and frequent multi-tasking with switching between tasks are likely to increase the overall cognitive load for the individual. The interaction between the individual and the digital world is uni-modal, consisting mainly of visual images of a limited size on a screen. There is a lack of integration of signals across the different sensory modules (vision, hearing, smell, touch, taste, etc.). This lack of integration may affect the representation of digital objects (a reduced number of dimensions in the representation). The experience is no longer linked to body sensation systems (embodiment). The screen is likely the limitation that shapes digital experiences.

Digitalization has also transformed social experiences. Compared with real-life social interactions, social exchanges through digital media enable the engagement with a much larger number of people, albeit in a much simpler manner. Social signals (e.g., 'likes' in social media such as the Facebook) are conveyed with the press of a button. People find it generally easier to interact digitally than in real life. However, negative interaction is also more likely to be countered online as it is perceived to have less direct consequences.

It is possible to create a digital self-identity on the online platform that is substantially different from the self-identity in real life as information such as gender and age are no longer verifiable. Easily manufactured self-identity is novel to human experience, and it creates new demands in theories of mind. The lack of real-life social encounters also means that empathic explications (see section 5.2.1) may be difficult. As a result, the representation of others may become simpler, and even dichotomous (good or bad). The resulting representation of the 'social group' (see section 6.4.7) may also become different structurally, with an increase in the number of individuals but a decrease in the number of dimensions for each individual. It would be more difficult to keep track of the shared information for sets of individuals in the group.

Digital objects comprise a new class of objects. They are informational rather than material. They are shared with others. Digital objects may represent real-life objects or they can be imaginary objects (such as cartoon characters). The mind separately keeps track of information from the real world and information from the imagined world. Emerging digital objects need to be tracked separately from the concrete real-life objects. Failure will result in a more diffuse boundary between the digital world and the material world, giving rise to a changed sense of reality.

There is some evidence that digitalization has led to a generation effect with deterioration in mental health (more loneliness, more suicidal ideation, more cognitive load) (Twenge, 2016). The observations are not yet conclusive as effects on a whole generation of young people growing up in the rapidly changing digital environment are difficult to demonstrate conclusively.

6.5 Motivation and Causality

Human experience takes place in a temporal stream. The basic structure of the mind has an intrinsic temporal dimension (see section 3.3 on the temporality of human experience).

Cognitions about the future, with probabilistic representations and action initiation, are handled separately from cognitions about the past, which have less probabilistic and re-combination possibilities. Probabilistic cognition is inherent to thinking about the future. Information is determined and fixed in the distant-past memory system (Bubic et al., 2010; Schacter et al., 2007; Tulving, 1985). At the confluence of the future and the past lie the perceptual and the action representations in the present moment.

Probabilistic systems allow for parallel searches for optimal solutions in response to a given input, using constraint satisfaction mechanisms (see Figure 6.9). Representation of future possibilities is similar to the tracking of a number of narrative accounts into the future. For future events there are possibilities to intentionally act in the present to steer towards a particular outcome (the narrative plot). The narrative structure stores information about the scenario and possible outcomes, with the given social information and constraints. This structure has a temporal dimension and it projects into the future to give predictions.

6.5.1   Temporal changes of states of mind

Evolving experience can be represented as a system that changes with time. The output (state of mind, SOM) of any one moment (Tn), SOM[Tn], will become part of the input of the next moment. SOM[T(n+1)]. The inputs for the next moment T(n+1) consist of the present environment ENV, the present state of mind SOM(T(n)), and long-term memory (LTM).

The outcome is monitored by the salience systems in the brain. Salience systems have the capacity to detect deviation from regularities, so that they learn to 'ignore' predictable regularities and engage with the unpredicted (i.e., salient) stimuli (Schacter et al., 2007; Smith et al., 2011). Regularity is predicted from current ENV patterns, encoded in short-term memory (STM prediction), as well as from information based on LTM and wider knowledge of the world (LTM prediction). These predictions form an anticipated state of mind and state of the world (expressed in the model as *anticipated* SOM[T(n+1)]). This anticipated state is compared with the actual state of the world SOM (T(n+1)). The discrepancy between the actual SOM[T(n+1)] and an *anticipated* SOM[T(n+1)] is calculated. If the discrepancy is above a threshold, a salience response is activated. This signifies the presence of significant unpredicted situations in the environment and directs the mind to engage and understand the novel situation.

Momentary representation of the contents of the mind has a basic structure: It contains components organized as the self and the environment. The environment

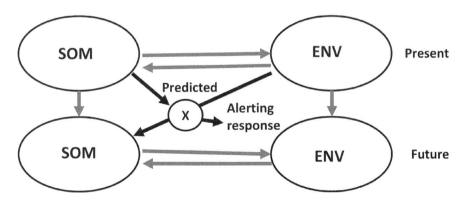

Figure 6.9. Predicted environment by state of mind (SOM) and the salience response. Current SOM together with the current environment (ENV) primes (points to) the predicted next SOM. When the actual next ENV is different from the predicted SOM, an alerting response is activated.

involves representations of people, of events, and of the world as a situational model (SOA) (Zwaan & Radvansky, 1998).

In modelling the temporal evolution of the network, a constraint satisfaction auto-associative network is a useful and parsimonious model. States of the network represent the process of resolving constraint satisfaction (CS) problems (Rumelhart et al., 1987b). The state of the constraint satisfaction network at any moment is characterized by the goodness-of-fit of the current network, given the external conditions (constraints) and the stored internal regularities. Such goodness-of-fit values can be quantified as energy levels (Amit, 1989). Each network state has a corresponding goodness-of-fit (energy) value. Collectively the energy values of all possible network states make up a two-dimensional surface called the 'energy landscape' (Amit, 1989). The location of the current network state amongst all possible state space will be determined by the 'constraint satisfaction' process. The current state is represented by a point in the energy landscape. It evolves with time along a direction amongst the entire 'state space' landscape so as to incrementally minimize the energy level (i.e., it tends to gravitate towards lower energy values on the surface; lower energy value is a signal of better goodness-of-fit). The shape of the energy landscape is itself dependent on the current state of the network. As the network evolves, the landscape changes and leads to the next state according to new constraints. Occasionally it will stay in a specific state for a longer period. This situation is described as an 'attractor'.

The SOM evolves either on its own (offline) or in association with inputs from the environment ENV (online). Changes in ENV can serve to renew SOM and dislodge it from stable configurations (local attractors), provided that sufficient 'noise' in the computation is allowed. A degree of noise (randomness in individual neuron behaviour) in the brain may thus be of functional value (Chen, 1994, 1995). The current SOM can influence the next SOM via the mechanism called 'priming' (i.e., introducing a 'bias' to influence the evolution of the network towards a particular solution). In our model, we consider the prefrontal cortex as a context-setting structure; that is it interacts with the posterior-cortex by providing activation (by focusing) on a certain part of the energy landscape and priming for a particular range of possible solutions.

6.5.2 Association between events

The flow between two ideas from one moment to the next can be more formally treated with a model.

Consider a set of nodes in the semantic net N1 . . . Nn, representing some aspect of the SOM at time 1 to time n, respectively. Each node N1, N2 . . . Nn is linked to a specific set of units (link N1 . . . n) in the net. N represents a semantic object with its meaning being derived from its relationship with other units. The connecting links contribute to the meaning of the nodes N1, N2, . . . Suppose N1 is linked to a set of nodes (linked N1) while N2 is linked to a different, partially overlapping, set of nodes (linked N2).

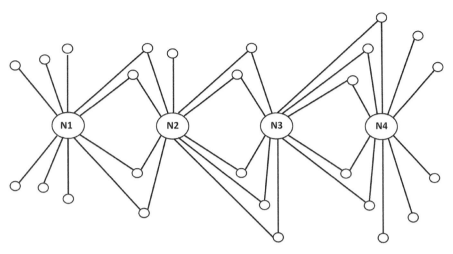

Figure 6.10. Sequential activation of an associative chain of ideas. How an idea N1 triggers via association the next idea N2? In the semantic net each node N1, N2, . . . is linked to a specific set of units in the net. After N1 is activated, the connecting links contribute to the activation of a set of related notes; one of them, N2, eventually 'wins' the activation competition and becomes the net content in the flow of subjective experience.

When N1 activation is followed by N2 activation in the next moment in time, N1 is considered to have provided a background for the activation of N2 through the co-activation of the linked N1 nodes. Linked N1 nodes, combined with the environmental input at the moment, as well as the input from long-term memory (such as personal propensities), results in the subsequent activation of the N2 node. At the end of the activation, the N2 and N1 nodes are both active (however, N1 will go into latency sooner, leaving N2 to be more active). The conjunction of N1N2 specifies a combined meaning more than N1 or N2 separately in determining the activation of N3. This chaining of immediate context thus determines the final output at a particular moment $Nt = f(aN(t-1)bN(t-2)cN(t-3)...)$, where a, b, c . . . are weights of decreasing influence for nodes of the more-distant past (see Figure 6.10). This is a model of how previous mental states influence the current mental state as if in a continuous stream. The stochastic nature of the effects is embedded in the probabilistic activation function of the individual units. The possibility for sudden change is enabled by the rich connectivity between units, enabling a catastrophe function to be present in parts of the energy landscape (see section 2.7.1). The dependence of the current states on the series of immediate past states provides a model for the context-dependences of SOM. In the psychopathological assessment of SOM it is important to consider the context provided by the immediately preceding states. The model highlights the importance of context in the clarification of mental symptoms.

6.5.3 Will and active direction

The human mind can actively exercise choice over the direction of thinking and in action. In computational terms this is implemented through keeping the activation of relevant units in the representation constant over time (clamping) of relevant units in the representation. Persistence of an activation pattern will influence action and thinking direction towards a particular path.

6.5.4 Motivation, planning, and goal-directed behaviour

Motivation involves the anticipation of the next SOM when there are several possible options. The option that is associated with the more 'desirable' outcome is calculated. Constraint satisfaction is applied to calculate the specific actions that will lead the external states towards the desired direction.

The next SOM(T+1)A, SOM(T+1)B, SOM(T+1)C are the *possible* states reachable within range from the current state, SOM(T). The AP difference between SOM(T) and SOM(T+1) represents what action needs to be carried out in order to arrive at that state.

The solution consists of identifying the AP schemata in the set of possible actions: SOM AP(A) AP(B) AP(C) etc., the one that will lead to SOM(T) evolving into the most desirable outcome, SOM(T+1)Mmax, the highest motivational value (Mmax). Likewise it also moves away from the undesirable outcome, that is, SOM(T+1)Mmin.

When there is a large incentive difference between the different outcomes SOM(T+1) (Mmax–Mmin), the stake of this action is high. This leads to a state of high arousal (high stake difference APdn) (see Figure 6.11).

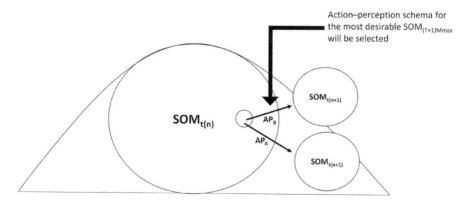

Figure 6.11. Motivation, planning, and goal-directed behaviour. State of Mind at time n, SOMt(n), contains a set of action-perception schema (APA, APB) leading to a set of potential next states, SOMt(n+1). Each of these states is associated with a reward value, the next state with the highest reward value along with its action-perception schema is chosen as the next goal-directed behaviour (see section 6.5.4).

When action is initiated, there is an agency signal involving an awareness of choice, the initiation, and ongoing monitoring, as the AP SOM unfolds with time. Critical to this process is the sense of control and the possibility of ongoing adjustment. This monitoring of an action is a crucial aspect of agency (Kühn et al., 2009).

The computation of motivational value can sometimes be high dimensional and may not be fully accessible to consciousness. Under these circumstances, it may correspond to the clinical observation of a 'somatic marker', which appears to awareness as a less definable 'intuition' (Damasio, 1994).

6.6 Basic Computations Acting on Representations

6.6.1 Constraint satisfaction

Constraint satisfaction is a general operation in neural networks that leads to a solution from a given set of initial conditions (Rumelhart et al., 1987b). It can be used as a generic model of computation processes in the brain/mind. Constraint satisfaction in mental operations can be expressed as moving from the initial starting set of objects + operation (e.g., [objects (A and B), operation (sum)] = constraint satisfaction (A+B)) to solution (A+B). Objects A, B, . . . can be semantic objects or operations (e.g., arithmetic or logical operations) (see Figure 6.12).

Constraint satisfaction operations move the state of the representation network towards a better overall 'coherence'. Each computation step in constraint satisfaction involves an incremental improvement in fit between the externally imposed conditions (activations) and internally stored regularities (connection weights). The energy landscape is a surface made up of points with energy levels corresponding to all the different possible activation states in the representation (i.e., different permutations of which unit is on and which unit is off amongst the population of neurons). In a network evolving in time, at any moment the particular network state is represented by a point in that 'state space' and its coherence (or energy) is represented by its height as located in the energy landscape surface. As the representation evolves with time, the point gravitates along a descending path on the energy landscape surface (better fit, lower energy). The energy level is a reflection of the overall goodness-of-fit of the representation at any one time. When an overall resolution is found, an energy minimum is reached. Constraint satisfaction presents a generic mechanism whereby a parallel distributed system can solve problems that involve multiple optimization requirements in a multi-dimensional state. The neuronal connectivity in the brain is optimally positioned to solve such problems. There are times when a quantum increase in goodness-of-fit is associated with a paradigm shift and adjustment of the cognitive model of the world.

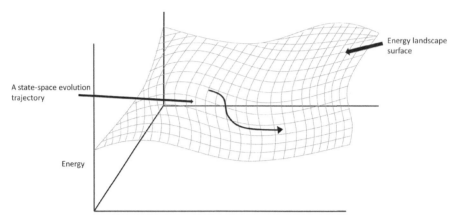

Figure 6.12. Constraint satisfaction in auto-associative networks. An auto-associative network consists of a population of connected nodes. The connections are specified by modifiable weights. Each possible state of the network (characterized by on-off status of each of the units) carries an energy value, depending on how the on-off states of units fit in with the connection weights patterns. Through interactive cycles of activations, the network gradually settles into an activity pattern that is consistent with the connection weights. This process is called constraint satisfaction, and can be represented in an 'energy landscape' diagram. In the diagram, energy value is represented in the vertical height. Different network states are represented by points in a surface with different heights (energy values). Activation change in a network is represented by a path on the map. According to constraint satisfaction rules, the path always follows a descending direction. The network arrives at a stable state when it reaches a local minimum, that is, a valley bottom that has a lower energy status than all surrounding points (see section 6.6.1).

6.6.2 External search-and-match operations

Searching operations for a target in the environment involves pattern recognition, screening, scanning, categorization, and exploration of new territorial space. It also involves the ability to zoom out occasionally to detect hidden patterns located at another scale level (see section 6.6.6 on zooming out).

6.6.3 Clamping and freeing operations

A series of learning during systematic explorations of the environment provides the content of the AP cycles (Fuster, 1990, 2002, 2004; Little & Sommer, 2011, 2013; Sommer & Wurtz, 2008; Swenson & Turvey, 1991; see section 5.1.2 on empathic explication). We shall apply the constraint satisfaction model to this process of mastering the environment.

Clamping-freeing operation

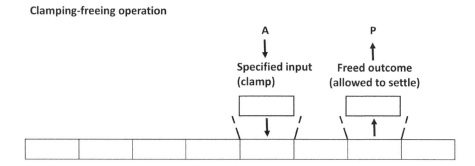

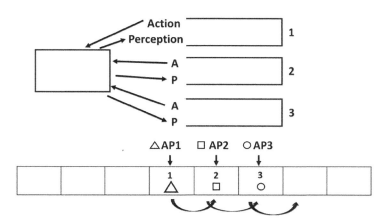

Figure 6.13. Clamping and freeing operations. In active exploration of an object, one can act upon the object to trigger responses and learn the relationships between actions and responses. In an uncontrolled situation many different actions can lead to different responses at the same time. It is difficult for the brain to work out causal relationships. More systematic exploration may involve clamping (making unchanged) all but one dimension (the freed dimension) and then use actions systematically to vary that dimension to observe the changes in response. Different dimensions in an object can be explored one by one through such action-perception cycles. The action-perception cycles (AP1, AP2, and AP3) bring forth a series of observations successively. The clamping-freeing system of exploration works by fixing most parameters and freeing only one parameter. This allows variations along that parameter to trigger different responses, learning of the mapping between action and response can then take place.

Explorations of the environment using the 'clamped' and 'freed' operation allow the learning to take place 'one dimension at a time'. This leads to a stepwise mastery of multi-dimensional models of the environment (see Figure 6.13). The approach involves clamping most variables so that they are fixed while allowing only one variable to be freed. Systematic variations (probing) in the single free variable are then made, resulting in different responses. The probe-response pairs drive learning over that dimension. After mastering one dimension, the explorations then shift to a new dimension. This approach is analogous to controlled empirical studies.

This approach reduces complex phenomena to a single dimension. Changes are predicted using the existing model. Prediction errors are used for the gradual learning of new input-output relationships in an updated model. When prediction error is minimized, the dimension is successfully mastered. The system then progresses to further explorations by freeing a new parameter in another dimension and then repeating the process. This process is repeated until all relevant dimensions have been explored.

Importantly, this model assumes that the input-output relationships in the different dimensions are independent of one another. This condition is assumed as the dimensions are explored independently. When interactions between two dimensions exist, it necessitates the exploration of the two dimensions simultaneously. There is a limit to the number of dimensions the mind can handle simultaneously in this manner. This limit is particularly severe as the interactions between dimensions are not always linear and incremental (see section 6.5.2). Higher dimensional non-linear patterns are better detected via different systems in the mind involving more parallel processing designs. Massively parallel systems appear to be able to robustly handle non-linear relationships between many variables (e.g., Rumelhart et al., 1987a).

The learning process described above is applicable to the exploration of a passive world (i.e., a one-person game, Colman, 2013). In the exploration of the social world involving 'intentional agents' a different system is required (see section 2.5.3). Knowledge involved in the modelling of intentions is indispensable (i.e., n-person games in game theory, Colman, 2013). Probabilistic computations with a high degree of tentativeness will have to be accommodated.

6.6.4 Convergent and divergent thinking

In a given representation, the ratio of clamped versus freed parameters in a constraint satisfaction process can result in different modes of processing (Rumelhart et al., 1987b).

The more knowledge is available, the more likely the mind will have sufficient information to solve a problem by a 'deductive' process. In deductive thinking (convergent thinking), the mind considers relevant possibilities from a universe based on known rules. Ruling out possibilities from the total universe is an important process in deduction. However, in order for top-down processes to rule out alternatives, the jigsaw puzzle needs to be in a state of near-completion. One needs a near-complete

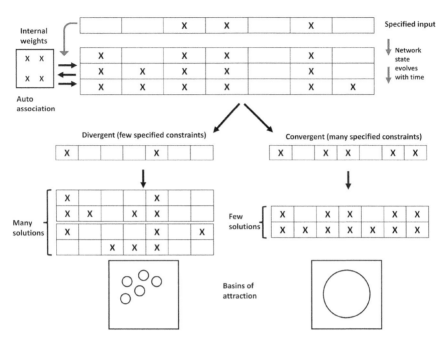

Figure 6.14. Convergent and divergent thinking in the constraint satisfaction model. Each step in constraint satisfaction evolves with time and moves towards more stable states (solutions). In divergent thinking, relatively few parameters are fixed (each step can potentially lead to more possible solutions). In convergent thinking, most of the parameters are already specified (fixed) (each step leads to fewer possible solutions). In the diagram, possible solutions are represented by basins of attraction (circles) in the energy landscapes (see section 6.6.4).

understanding of all relevant variables. A reasoning space in which the information is far from complete is not a good platform for deductive (constraint satisfaction) processing. Deductive (convergent) thinking involves the clamping of parameters in most of the dimensions in the representation, allowing only a few free parameters. Convergent thinking is common in goal-directed problem-solving attempts.

In contrast, divergent thinking fixes only a few parameters and uses a larger proportion of free parameters. Divergent thinking generates a wide range of creative ideas (see Figure 6.14). An example of divergent thinking is to 'think of all possible alternative uses of an empty can'.

6.6.5 Autonomous representations

Constraint satisfaction in TOM tasks can take place in two modes: (1) an effortful rational mode and (2) an autonomous spontaneous mode. The effortful mode uses convergent problem solving. The autonomous mode adopts a divergent mode of operation. Autonomous settling is particularly important where a large number of parameters need to be considered in order to allow the TOM representation to approximate real-life predictions. In the autonomous mode, other's TOM representation is given a free rein to evolve to arrive at its own predictions. There is minimal explicit control from the rational conscious self.

6.6.6 Zooming-out operation (enlargement of constraint space)

Different representations can share overlapping feature dimensions (e.g., the dimension of 'colour' may be shared by the representations of 'animals' and 'food'). The set of dimensions involved in a given processing is assembled at the time of the processing. The number of dimensions involved in the operation can define the size of representations. When more dimensions are involved, more variables are processed in larger representations. When fewer dimensions are involved, a more focused consideration of fewer parameters is involved. It is possible for the number of involved dimensions to change during processing. When the number of dimensions reduces, a more focused operation with fewer units is deployed. This 'zooming in' process occurs when the subject 'focuses' to generate a solution to a part of the problem. When a larger number of dimensions are involved, the subject steps back to consider a wider range of possible options. Such 'zooming out' thinking process involves a broadening of the constraint space (see Figure 6.15). Zooming out is a key component in creative processes such as

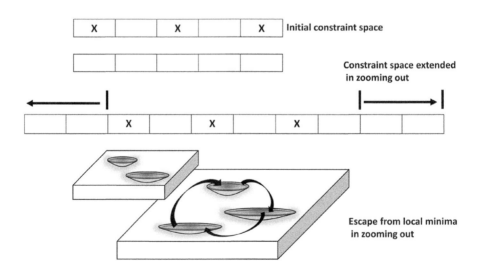

Figure 6.15. Zooming out (enlargement of constraint space). When alternative solutions are required, we may step-back to consider a wider range of options. Accordingly, the processing unit expands to include more dimensions in its consideration. This is the 'zooming out' (out of the box) lateral thinking process (see section 6.6.4).

lateral thinking (de Bono, 1970), divergent thinking (Hocevar, 1980), humour perception (Forabosco, 1992; Suls, 1983) and bi-association (Koestler, 1964).

6.7 Mental Operations from a Representational Perspective

Having considered the nature of a set of basic computational operations that may
mediate cognitive experiences, it is helpful to suggest a minimalist list of basic cognitive
processes that underlie human subjective experiences. This non-exhaustive list is kept
to a minimum by conceptually decomposing candidate processes into their component
parts. These processes are the common building blocks of daily human experiences.
Many complex experiences can be constructed from these basic building blocks. We
list these processes to facilitate considerations of how their failure may contribute to
psychopathological phenomena (see Chapter 7).

1. Perception

Receiving sensory information from the environment. Top-down interaction already
occurs in perception. Top-down processing is essential for improving signals in a noisy
environment.

2. Resting

AP loops consist of units in which perception is closely coupled with action (Hommel,
2001; Turvey & Fitzpatrick, 1993). The most basic of this is simple instrumental learning cycles. Learning takes place in unfamiliar environments and leads to mastery of
the environment. In a familiar environment, highly predictable AP loops may take up
much of the waking experience. An example of a highly predictable resting AP cycle
is auto-contact behaviour (such as scratching; Morris, 1978). In auto-contact behaviour, the results are fully predictable and there is no information for active learning.
Closed AP loops fill much of the time of basic resting existence. Recent imaging studies
suggest that this state might be associated with specific resting patterns of brain activities (Callard & Margulies, 2014). While there is little engagement with novel information in the environment, the brain in this state may be performing important internal
re-organization of information (see section 6.4.9 on daydreaming).

3. Monitoring

Monitoring involves observation, with the prediction of expected states in the environment (this can take place at the same time as AP loops; see section 6.5.3). Deviations
from the normal expectations will alert the salience system. This alert is likely mediated
by dopamine.

4. Exploring

The exploring state involves searching for a novel target in the environment. The search
may lead to exploratory activities and the mastery of new aspects of the environment.

5. Recall

Recall involves active retrieval from memory of remembered representations.

6. Imagining

Imagining is the use of mental representation to conceptualize not-yet-in-existence SOA. This can result from re-combination of components from existing SOA. This counterfactual ability (counterfactual thinking, Deacon, 1997; also see section 6.2.1; Roese, 1994) to represent SOA not actually in existence is important for imagination, planning, deception, and social communication (see section 6.4).

7. Problem solving

In convergent thinking, most parameters of a situation are known. The objective is to search for an unknown parameter based on the current known input and the internal model of the situation. Initial definition of the search space is specified by defining the dimensions involved. Effort is made to minimize unnecessary or irrelevant dimensions. The outcome is a solution to the problem that maximally satisfies the external and internal constraints.

8. Zooming out

Zooming out consists of thinking creatively out of the (current) 'box', involving the consideration of a broader contextual framework not previously considered. Zooming in consists of reducing the dimensions under consideration in order to arrive at a focused solution.

9. Actively willed actions

A person can apply a sustained intention (will) to initiate and maintain particular actions. This leads to an experience of voluntary choice. This also includes active choice for the direction of conscious engagements with particular contents. In making a choice, it is also necessary to negate other choices and not to go into alternative directions (inhibition, suppression of distractions)

10. Empathy

Empathy involves thinking about what others might be experiencing. Empathy involves the use of the capacity to estimate the mental states of other individuals and is a fundamental capability that underlies social communication.

11. Pointing

Pointing is the action of communicating to another person by referring to an external object so that the attention of the other person is drawn to the object (Tomasello & Call, 1997; Tomasello et al., 2005). It is a distinctive human action. Gestural pointing establishes a shared external world. A toddler will be able to point by 18 months. It constitutes the basis of referring. Awareness of 'being pointed at' forms the basis of self-concept development. Language is developed as a more sophisticated pointing action essentially based on gestural physical pointing.

12. Linguistic narration

This involves the narration of verbal propositional-based statements about the world to communicate a version of the SOA to other individuals. The reception of a propositional SOA leads to updating one's own SOA model of the world. Communication of social SOA is an important action to define social groups and cooperation in human life.

7

Representation Failure and Psychopathology

The current account makes explicit the role of representations in mediating experiences. It enables the potential considerations of psychopathological phenomena as failures of representation. We explicate the basic operations in representations using the simplest parallel distributed model (see section 6.5.4). We explore potential mechanisms in which representational processes can fail and illustrate how these may be relevant for understanding human psychopathological experiences. We also explain how information computation failure in the human brain can give rise to the qualitative characteristics of a wide range of psychopathological phenomena. It is important to note that this chapter tries to explicate anomalous phenomena as much as possible by referring to the potential processes involved in mental representation. We do not make claims that the account is exhaustive. However, it is important to appreciate the limits of explanation given what we already know. Making these explicit leads to new perspectives and new ways of thinking about psychopathological mechanisms. This account does not claim to be the final say. It recognizes itself as part of a process of increasing the understanding of psychopathological processes.

It is worth noting the traditional distinction between positive and negative aspects of psychopathology. Negative processes are the impaired functioning of normal mechanisms, representing a loss of normal processes. Positive processes are an anomalous presence of pathology. They are generally more difficult to account for. Traditional accounts often propose failure of inhibition of latent processes (Crow, 1980, 1982; Jackson, 1932). A representational perspective offers explanatory possibilities to understand a range of positive psychopathology.

7.1 Constraint Satisfaction Failures

7.1.1 Context failure (clamping)

In the constraint satisfaction (CS) model, a problem is solved by evoking the external conditions as 'givens' (clamped constraints) and then allowing the free parameters in the representational network to settle into a solution based on internal regularities. CS failure results from a failure to regulate the 'clamping-freeing' process, that is, clamping

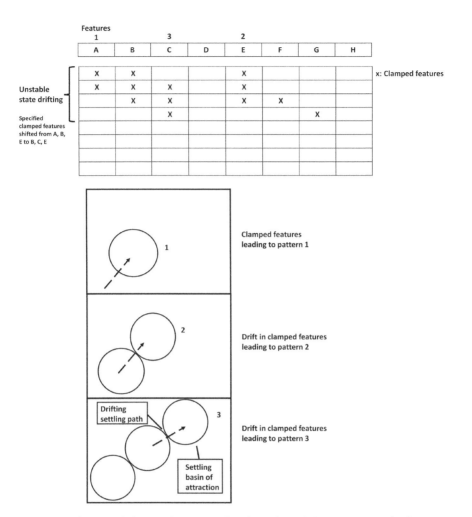

Figure 7.1. Clamping failure and context-related psychopathology. Contextual information for a representation is contained in the relevant associated dimensions. For that information to be made relevant to the processing in the representation, the contextual dimensions need to be kept activated (clamped, indicated by 'x', on features A, B, and E) during the operation. When this process fails a number of dysfunctions may arise. Above: normal contextual influence on processing; Middle: failure in clamping may lead to loss of contextual influence on the current processing (middle); Below: weak or transient clamping leading to drifting of context over time away from original context (clamped features became C and E over time) (see section 7.1.1).

of some feature units for just long enough to allow the rest to freely evolve. If clamping is too rigid, the processing may be restricted by the inflexible context. If the clamping is too feeble, the context may drift too readily for a stable solution to emerge. Clamping failure can offer a computational perspective in understanding pathological phenomena such as thought disorganization (tangential thinking) and perseveration (insufficient clamping) (see Figure 7.1). Dysregulated clamping results in maladjustments in shifting, either in drifting contexts or fixed rigid contexts.

7.1.2 Signal synchronization failure

Neural synchronization is an important mechanism for maintaining the coherence of information relating to individual objects across multiple processing streams (Singer, 2000). In the brain, information that originates from a single object is eventually handled by a number of parallel streams. It is important to have some means of tracking which information belongs to a given object, particularly if a number of objects are being processed at the same time. It appears that the neural signals relating to a single object are oscillating in-phase, even when segregated into different processing streams in different parts of the brain (see Figure 7.2). These oscillations are of relatively high frequency (detected in the gamma-band in electroencephalography). Failure of gamma-band synchronization in psychosis has been postulated to result in anomalous coherence as well as inadequate coherence in representations, giving rise to positive and negative symptoms, respectively (Phillips & Silverstein, 2003; Silverstein & Keane, 2011; Uhlhaas & Singer, 2010). In terms of mental representations, the different dimensions in a representation (location, size, texture, movement, etc.) are processed by different brain systems. The information is linked to a single object in the environment by

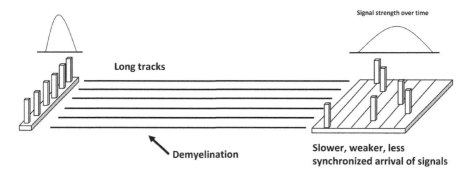

Figure 7.2. Long-tract conduction failure. Parallel signals along longer neural tracts may become desynchronized. This may involve a lowering of signal conduction efficiency (e.g., in inefficient myelination), resulting in increase in variability in conduction speed on top of slowing. In parallel distributed processing, less synchronization in the arrival of signals to the next set of processing units will affect the strength and clarity of the set of arriving signals (see section 7.1.2).

gamma-band synchronization processes. Failure in these processes results in a representation with weakened structure; that is, the dimensions hang together only loosely.

The failure of synchronization can also arise from a number of other mechanisms. Synaptic events and modulation by excitatory and inhibitory cortical pathways are possible candidates. In addition, neural conduction along long tracts in the brain may take a finite amount of time. Parallel signals along long tracts may become temporally diffused (desynchronized) if the axonal conduction processes are compromised (e.g., by demyelination). Such impediments result not only in a slowing of signal conduction but, importantly, in an increase in variability in the conduction velocity between individual fibres, resulting in reduced synchronization in the arrival of signals to the next set of processing units (Miller, 2008). Lengthening of reaction times with increased variabilities in various brain domains is an observation frequently made in schizophrenia, affecting phenomena such as motor reaction time and event-related potentials. Synchronization failure weakens the definition and sharpness of signals and compromises computations such as CS in a general manner (see section 7.1.2.1).

7.1.2.1 *Generic constraint satisfaction failure*

General CS failure can occur even where simple generic mechanistic processes are involved. An example is the effects on simple reaction time tasks when a lengthening of response time and a decrease in accuracy of response are observed. This generic CS failure can contribute to reduced information handling efficiency in a broad range of cognitive areas.

7.1.2.2 *Constraint satisfaction threshold shifts*

Computations in propositional thinking necessitate a flexible range of CS threshold to be adjusted based on particular contexts. The CS threshold determines the level of coherence required before CS processing is considered resolved. For instance, in poetry, a more diffused mode of operation calls for a lower CS threshold than for rational thinking, such as in computer programming.

The CS threshold may also be programmed to change with time. Problem solving can start with a less stringent criterion (lower requirement for CS fit) for an initial direction. This is followed by a gradual tightening of the criteria (higher requirement for fit). This process is called 'simulated annealing'. It may lead to efficient solutions in a limited amount of time (Rumelhart et al., 1987).

In situations of dopamine excess, salience would lead to a pressing search for expected CS resolutions. As a result, a loosening in CS threshold may be involved. To accommodate a broader range of observations, the system also searches more widely for patterns with more parameters involved and to arrive more readily at possible solutions. This situation may be relevant to the experiences of ideas of reference and spurious salience in psychotic states.

7.2 Lateral Inhibition Failures

Cortical inhibitory processes help not only to modulate overall activation levels but specifically to provide contrast enhancement in representations (Murray et al., 2006). Cortical GABA interneurons play an important role in these processes. Failure in contrast processing may result in representations becoming fuzzier and less distinctive (see Figure 7.3). Failure in cortical inhibitory mechanisms has been implicated in a number of conditions. For example, recent evidence suggests failure in contrast processing in the working memory as well as the visual system in patients with psychosis (Serrano-Pedraza et al., 2014).

7.3 Top-down Priming Biases

Information arriving from the external world is processed in stages along the lines of incoming perceptual processing streams. Raw sensory information about the world is analysed and patterns are recognized at each stage. The output from one stage of processing becomes the input to the next stage. The information flows from earlier sensory

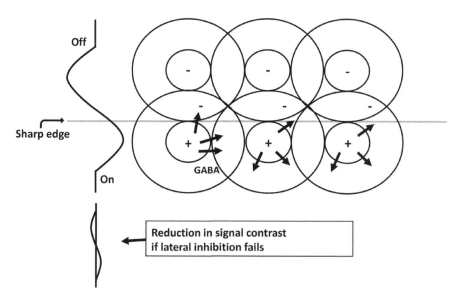

Figure 7.3. Lateral inhibition and contrast enhancement failure. Cortical neurons in the visual systems (and possibly other systems) not only excite the target neurons but also inhibit unrelated neurons close to the target neurons (lateral inhibition). In the visual system this results in sharper boundaries of the resulting signal, serving a contrast enhancement function. It is possible that such function is served not only in the spatial perceptual system but also in cognitive systems such as working memory. GABA interneurons are probably involved in the lateral inhibition functions. Failure in contrast processing may result in less distinctive and effective signals (see section 7.2).

information (bottom) to more processed information at higher levels (top). Each stage of processing involves matching the current information with existing templates from memory. Top-down influences involve the higher-level patterns driving activation of expected patterns at a lower level. This is important for the handling of noisy and incomplete information in real life. Top-down 'expectations' thus 'prime' or 'bias' the detection of the expected stimuli from incoming information. The final percept is completed through combined bottom-up and top-down processing (see Figure 7.4).

7.4 Catastrophe Dynamics

A system may exhibit a catastrophe dynamic when there is a sudden state change along one dimension as a result of a gradual variation in other dimensions (catastrophe theory, Thom, 1972/1975). A typical catastrophe can be visualized in three dimensions with axes x, y, and z (see Figure 7.5). We consider when z is fixed at a certain value, there is a continuous sigmoidal function between x and y, so that a small increase in x is associated with a small increase in y (line a, figure 7.5). At another value for z, however, the relationship between x and y is described by a hysteresis (line b, figure 7.5). A small increase in x at the threshold value results in a large jump in y. However, once in the region of a high y, a reduction in x does not result in a return to a lower y at the same threshold. Y will return to a lower level only at a lower x. Such hysteresis dynamics occur in many natural phenomena, such as the relationship between volume and pressure in the pulmonary alveoli.

A model of catastrophe dynamics for prison disturbance may serve to illustrate the role of interaction between component units (Zeeman, 1977). In this model z represents the 'extent of interaction between different inmates', x represents 'dissatisfaction', and y represents 'prison unrest'. When there is little inmate interaction, dissatisfaction increases with unrest in a linear fashion, but with more interaction between inmates, mutual influence between inmates becomes an additional factor and a sharper rise in unrest at a critical threshold is encountered. Increase in dissatisfaction results in a hysteresis, with more repression of the dissatisfaction at low dissatisfaction levels, but a flip takes place at the threshold when there is a critical level of dissatisfaction. It is worth noting that after this transition, simple reduction of dissatisfaction is not sufficient to reduce the unrest. It may be necessary to reduce the z-axis value (i.e., by restricting communication) before reduction in dissatisfaction has a better chance to work. The dynamics of sudden changes in the mind/brain can be considered with a model similar to the prison unrest catastrophe by virtue of its strongly interconnected units. In this system the interconnectedness of semantic units is analogous to communication between individuals in the prison unrest model and constitute the z-axis. In a highly interconnected state, a more bi-phasic behaviour of the network is exhibited, resulting in the possibility of sudden phase transition. In a less interconnected state a more linear incremental change results in a gradual development of abnormalities: Y-axis represents pathological behaviour, and x-axis represents the pro-illness factor (such

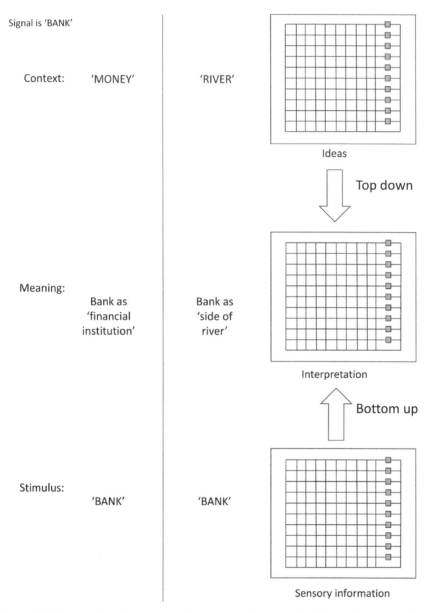

Figure 7.4. Excessive top-down processing can result in errors in interpreting signals from the environment. This can occur in the presence of weak bottom-up signals (as in sensory deprivation) or overactive top-down signals (as in intense anticipation of specific targets, e.g., in grief). Top-down processing disorders can result in illusions, hallucinations, and delusions. It is important to note that top-down disorders may result in hallucinations in all sensory modalities (e.g., visual, tactile, auditory, olfactory, gustatory modalities, etc.). The pathological mechanisms in top-down hallucinations may be different from those involved specifically in verbal hallucinations (see section 7.3 on the inner speech hypothesis).

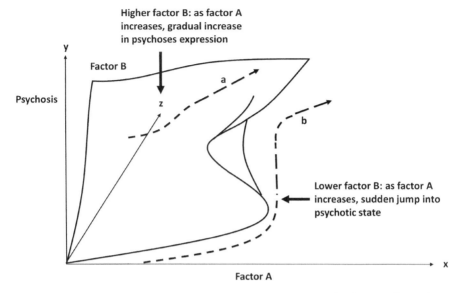

Figure 7.5. Catastrophe theory of symptom onset. Using the example of onset of a psychotic episode, in a gradual onset expression of psychosis. At higher factor B levels, when there is a small increase in factor A, there will be a small increase in psychosis. At lower factor B levels, when there is a small increase in factor A at a threshold value, there can be a large jump in psychosis. Factor B is crucial in determining the behaviour of the temporal relationship between factor A and the outcome (see section 7.4).

as genetics or dopamine abnormality). We note that x is not restricted to one single dimension, and further factors can be accommodated in a multi-dimensional catastrophe model. This model helps us to conceptualize how sudden state transitions can result from continuous changes along a number of other dimensions. We can use this model to interpret the mode of illness onset as suggesting the presence or otherwise of an underlying catastrophe phenomenon. This model can therefore help us to focus our efforts to identify the x and z dimensions in understanding the illness and predicting the response to treatment. For instance, it may be necessary to address the z-axis as well as the x-axis in treatment. In the case of psychosis, the z-axis may involve connectivity in the cortical network that normally detects salience and eventually drives dopamine response. Dopamine activity can be located in the x-axis, with the y-axis representing psychotic experiences.

7.5 Spurious Attractors

The term 'spurious attractor' refers to the emergence of novel representations not previously encountered in the network. The retrieved pattern does not correspond to any previously encountered patterns (memories) (see Figure 7.6b). A spurious attractor is

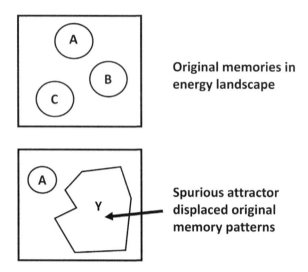

Original memories in
energy landscape

Spurious attractor
displaced original
memory patterns

Figure 7.6a. Spurious attractor and memory saturation. In the state space of a parallel distributed processing model, stable states (attractors A, B, and C) represent states that are possible stable 'solutions' the system may finally rest in. They usually correspond to previous patterns that the system has been exposed to (memories). However, under certain conditions 'spurious' attractors (Y) may arise. Spurious attractors are large stable states that do not correspond to previous patterns (see section 7.5).

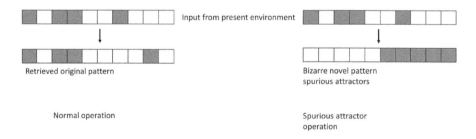

Input from present environment

Retrieved original pattern

Bizarre novel pattern
spurious attractors

Normal operation

Spurious attractor
operation

Figure 7.6b. Operation of representation under spurious attractors. Left upper rows: input from present environment. Bottom rows: retrieved memory pattern, which corresponds to the previous memory. Right input from present environment does not retrieve a close pattern from memory but retrieves a totally unrelated pattern (see section 7.5).

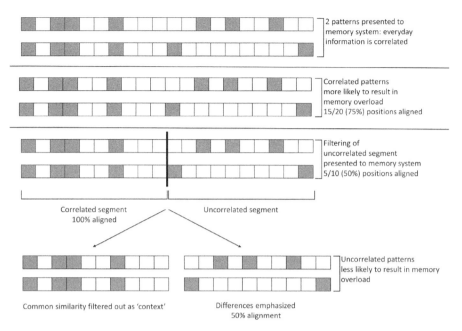

Figure 7.6c. Correlated input patterns, spurious attractor, and filtering. Top: Attempts to store correlated patterns are more likely to challenge memory limits and result in memory overload. Overloaded memory may predispose to the appearance of spurious attractors. Bottom: Parsing the incoming information into an invariant component and a distinctively varying component enhances the differences between input patterns (orthogonalization). The invariant component serves as contextual space. The varying component is the foreground. This arrangement can reduce memory overload in the foreground (see section 7.5).

an emergent phenomenon in that it arises in networks under certain computational conditions (see Figure 7.6a). A *de novo* (entirely new) pattern is encountered in the process. It has no correspondence to previous encountered regularities. Spurious attractors thus lead to a new representation that has never been seen before, and one that can violate previous regularities.

Spurious attractors emerge when the memory capacity of a computational network is overloaded. In a generic model for associative memory, it has been found that given a certain network size, the number of memories that can be stored is finite. The capacity for memory storage also depends on the distinctiveness of the patterns. Optimal capacity occurs when the patterns are perfectly uncorrelated (or as vectors, 'orthogonalized'). Memory performance declines when patterns become correlated (Amit, 1989) (see Figure 7.6c).

The formation of theory of mind (TOM) and community of mind (COM) (see section 6.2.2) imposes a heavy cognitive load on the mind (in real life TOM is often not fully implemented, Keysar et al., 2003). There is much individual variation in the capacity for TOM and COM. TOM and COM representations require the computationally intensive speculation of other people's perspective. Cognitive economy is attained—only to some extent—by grouping individuals (i.e., stereotyping, Sherman et al., 2011).

When an associative computational system operates near to its capacity, overloading of the system may lead to spurious attractor memories. It has been pointed out that spurious attractors in computational systems bear computational resemblance to features that may correspond to the formation of delusions in the mind (violate known regularities, do not correspond to known memories) (Amit, 1989; Chen, 1994, 1995; Hoffman & McGlashan, 1993).

In real life, incoming stimuli (daily perceptual experiences) are highly correlated (they share many features). The memory system has to adapt to the common occurrence of repetitive features and the rare occurrence of novel features. The system is more prone to saturation when patterns to be remembered are correlated (Amit, 1989). It is more demanding for a system to store recall patterns that are similar (correlated) because of a greater level of interference between patterns. One computation strategy to reduce overloading is to emphasize the novel features and de-emphasize common repetitive features.

Processing to extract novel features from the environment might be a function of the hippocampus (Chen, 1995; Eichenbaum et al., 1996; Rolls, 1996). The computation may involve 'orthogonalization' of incoming feature patterns to highlight the differences and downplay the similarities. This involves a 'similarity-difference' operation in the brain to parse the repeated contextual information from the distinctive foreground information.

The appearance of spurious attractors has been utilized to model the psychopathological appearance of novel output and is one of the few cognitive science models that offer an account of not only a reduced output (which is possible in many models) but also the emergence of an anomalous output (which is rarely successfully modelled). Spurious attractors offer a unique account for bizarre contents of psychopathological phenomena (Chen, 1994, 1995; Hoffman & McGlashan, 1993). A further account of 'strange' content is the 'latent computational fragments' (see section 7.6 and Figure 7.7).

Some time ago a patient reported an experience of hearing a dog barking in Cantonese. We can consider the experience in representational terms. The experience has the usual dimensions involved in auditory perception, with vividness, external sources localization, lack of control, and so forth. The unusual combination is the co-existence of two voice characteristic dimensions, that of a barking noise and of a linguistic-content dimension. In addition, these features are not just co-existing but are blended together to produce a unitary auditory stream. These features render the experience structurally anomalous. The representation structure is fundamentally changed. It is not just an anomaly in the individual dimension, but different dimensions that normally are incompatible are aggregated. This hallucinatory experience has a 'bizarre quality' similar to 'bizarreness' in delusions. In conventional psychopathology 'bizarreness' is used to describe delusions but is seldom used for hallucinations. With a representational analysis, there is a rationale for including the dimension of 'bizarreness' for hallucinations.

7.6 'Latent' Computational Fragments

7.6.1 Semantic and emotive fragments

In the process of absorbing information, some relatively intact fragments of representation may co-aggregate in computation. Fragments as units that co-segregate may not necessarily have an inherent meaning or distinctive function. They may consist of ideational, cognitive, or emotive features, or their combinations. They could be re-deployed as discrete units in future computations.

These fragments are 'sub-symbolic' (Smolensky, 1995). They do not necessarily have distinctive identities. They are less communicable by linguistic propositions and are often not accessible to the conscious mind.

The more meaningful of these fragments can sometimes be named. Once linked with a name, it opens up better possibilities of interacting in mutuality with other semantic units. With mutual support from other semantic units, they can inherit a life of their own. That existence can become relatively independent of the original sources. These fragments may be encountered in psychopathology as 'repeated' themes, both as psychotic and as obsessive-compulsive symptoms.

7.6.2 'Strange representations' in semantic corners

When links are formed internally in the semantic net between two nodes (both with external references), new internal nodes can be formed without input from external objects. In this situation, the two nodes can be linked to one another as well as to a third internal node. Together they can influence the convolutions in the adjacent semantic space, without additional external referent (see Figure 7.7 and section 7.1). This is the sphere of the inner world, the realm of magical imagination. They are unlike bizarre representations in that they do not defy existing semantic relationships. Bizarre representations violate existing semantic relationships. Thus there are two different kinds of imaginary representations: one is congruent with semantic rules, and the other violates them. The discriminating test would be to see if the idea is understandable by others. If it is understandable, this is an indication that there is likely congruence with the population-shared semantic world. The assessment of understandability is fundamental to psychopathological assessments (Jaspers, 1913/1963).

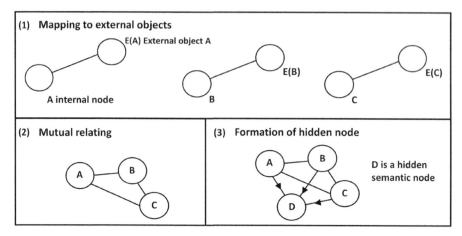

Figure 7.7. Hidden semantic corners. (1) Mapping to external nodes: Internal semantic notes (A, B, and C) link with objects in the empirical external world (E(A) E(B), and E(C)). (2) Semantic links are formed internally in the net between the nodes (A, B, and C); (3) Mutual relating: The internal nodes (A, B, and C) are linked to one another as well as to a third, entirely internal, node (D). D is a hidden semantic node (see section 7.6).

8

Towards a New Representational Framework in Psychopathology

Classical descriptive psychopathology has divided symptoms into groups corresponding to an implicit classification of healthy psychological functions (e.g., memory, language, attention, and perception, as in Fish & Hamilton, 1985). However, whether this conventional grouping of mental functions is an optimal description of the human mind is a question not yet fully examined.

In an ancient Chinese metaphor, a butcher is known for his exceptional skills in cutting meat. Someone asked whether his secret lies in the extraordinary sharpness of his blades. The butcher responded: there is a natural pattern in everything. If one goes against the natural patterns, every task becomes difficult. If one goes along the natural patterns, every task is easy. The art of the butcher does not lie in the sharpness of the blade but in knowing the natural organization of the body. Being able to discern the ways in which things are organized in nature will make a difference to the efficacy in understanding it.

Grouping of psychopathology based on conventional psychological functions is not without *a priori* assumptions. Conventional assumptions about psychological functions implicitly follow a division of mental phenomena based upon conventional computer technology, yielding domains such as perception, central executive, working memory, and long-term memory. It should not be taken for granted that these are necessarily the best way to dissect mental functions.

In seeking a more comprehensive framework for psychopathology, we explore a broader but coherent perspective using (1) 'representation' as a common framework and (2) considerations from evolutionary psychology.

This broader perspective affords a re-grouping of psychological processes and new conceptualization of their possible disturbances. The following is a list of the major groups of psychopathology categories suggested from such an approach. We shall start with disorders to do with 'relating'. Under this group there are problems with 'general relating', 'affective relating', and 'relating to inner representations'. The second group of disorders involves the ability to voluntarily initiate choices and actions. The third group of disorders is located in the domain of mental representations of other peoples: it includes some innovative perspectives arising directly from the current approach, including disorders of automaticity and compartmentalization. Finally, we consider disorders of interaction between representations, such as failure in consolidation of memory or in contextual influence. The psychopathological modules proposed in the current thesis cut across conventional categories in psychopathology. For instance, hallucinations will be divided into two distinct types, one to do with aberrant top-down processing, the other to do with aberrant automaticity (or a loss of agency) in inner 'models of others' in the social world. Likewise, the traditional category of a delusion is probably too broad and heterogeneous. In the current approach, disorders of top-down processing, agency, mental representations of other peoples, addressing, and compartmentalization of information can contribute to different phenomena that are currently all grouped under the single category of 'delusion'.

8.1 Disorders of Relating

A key phenomenological feature in human subjective experience is 'relating'. Relating can be directed to the world, to others, to things, to ideas or to oneself. It is useful to group pathological conditions in which this basic act of relating is compromised. Relating can fail in a general way. It can also fail in a content-specific manner (e.g., natural objects, others, ideas, self). We recognize that relating to internally generated ideas can also potentially become dysfunctional.

8.1.1 Disorder of general relating to external environment

In a generalized lowering of engagement with the external environment, representations are weakened and feebly linked to external objects. This general failure of engagement with all objects in the mind corresponds to the acute confusional state (or delirium) in conventional psychopathology. It is important to recognize this state as it indicates a widespread systemic brain failure typically suggesting the presence of general medical conditions (such as hypoxia, septicaemia, CVA, or encephalitis). Investigations and treatment of the underlying physiological failure are indicated.

8.1.2 Disorders of excessive relating

Of the many stimuli in the environment, a person has to adaptively choose which stimuli to engage with. This choice involves higher cognitive decisions that take into consideration the past experiences as well as motivational factors. Some pathological processes compromise the ability to select relevant stimuli. The person may end up responding inappropriately to whatever stimulus is presented in front of him, regardless of the situation. Patients with such 'environmental dependency syndrome' (see also section 8.4.4, Lhermitte, 1986) cannot help responding to any object placed in front of him by picking it up and then using it (utilization behaviour), no matter how inappropriate the context is. For example, during the clinical interview, when a spectacle is placed on the desk, the patient will pick up the spectacles and put it on, even though they do not belong to him and it does not help his eyesight.

8.1.3 Disorders of affective relating

Affective features are universally embedded in all representations. Emotions may also constitute discrete representations. Affective dimensions and representations are closely integrated with perceptual or interpretative representations and establish priming interactions with them (see Figure 8.1). A theory of how the interaction between these domains takes place in delusions has been proposed (Stein & Ludik, 1998). In this framework the representations in the mind are categorized into three groups: perceptual, interpretative, and affective. Perceptual information is received from sensory organs. It provides input to interpretative networks. The interpretative network computes a state of affairs (SOA) for the current situation based on incoming perceptual information. The interpretative network and the perceptual network are linked to the affective network. The affective network arrives at an affective state based on the incoming information from the perceptual and the interpretative networks. These influences are bidirectional. The affective network provides top-down input to prime the interpretative network and the perceptual networks in a direction congruent with the affect state. The interpretative network also provides priming to the perceptual network and biases the interpretation of sensory information to a direction congruent with the current SOA. Each of the networks integrates incoming bottom-up information with top-down priming information to arrive at a stable state.

Affect can be positive or negative and is thus 'directional'. Handling the emotionally positive and negative representations in the mind involves differential responses. Representations associated with negative affect are distanced from awareness. This may involve evolutionarily relevant stimulus (objects associated with blood or dirt,

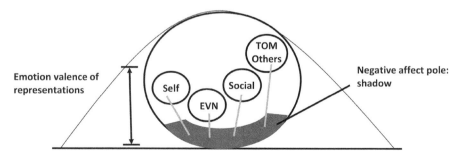

Figure 8.1. Affective processing of negative representations in the mind. Self, environment, social, and theory of mind of Others may be attached to negative affect, as shown as grey shadow. The lines represent affective distances from a representation to the negative semantic pole (see section 8.1.3).

trypophobic objects with multiple holes, etc.). Selective distancing from these objects facilitates survival. Even in modern life, representations associated with negative affect are often distanced from awareness. This distance may become more distorted in the effective sterile modern digital world.

How are these negative representations segregated in the mind? We propose that there are informational regions that are more distanced from immediate daily awareness. These regions accommodate representations that are associated with unwelcomed emotions (see Figure 8.1).

It is necessary for the mind to handle these negative affective feature dimensions effectively. Otherwise they may result in unforeseen effects that override other representations. If negative affect is attached to self-representations, it results in negative self-feelings. This situation may be encountered in psychopathological conditions such as depressive disorders and borderline personality disorder.

If negative affective features are attached to external representations, it may result in phobia, obsessive-compulsive symptoms, or persecutory ideations. In psychodynamic theory, such externally attached negative affect is described as 'projection' (Samuels, 1985).

It is important to reflect upon the nature of the 'I' in the basic experiential unit (see section 3.4). The mind is inhabited by the diverse interests and directions of its different components. The 'I' component is not a unitary entity. Our model of man's subjective experience enables us to appreciate that the 'self' is only part of the whole in the basic experiential unit (see section 3.4). A healthy integrated 'self' enhances the prospects of actualizing latent potentials in the individual.

We can refer to the less accessible representations as being located in a 'psychological bladder space'. It is the area in which the negative representations distanced from the conscious mind reside. When ideas do not pass through the censorship of the filter, they are deposited into this 'psychological bladder'. These distanced experiences may be displaced to other representations (of other persons or things). This 'psychological bladder' has a role to play in 'cleaning up' the canvas of consciousness. The representational 'bladder' is important for psychological well-being. Like the physiological bladder, it is a necessary organ for the exchanges between the internal and external worlds. Space for handling unwanted information discarded from the construction of the highly organized life of the mind is important. In the mind, informational waste products are created in a person in the pursuit of positive goals, growth, maturation, and orderliness. The waste products are handled in the psychological bladder space.

Dysfunctions of the psychological bladder space include significant information leakage to other objects, leading to the building up of an excessive self-dislike or dislike of some aspects of the world, and displacement of negative feelings towards representations of other persons. Net excess in negative contents may result in a free-floating surge in negative feelings and/or aggression, which may seek release relentlessly. The psychological bladder needs to be managed so as not to overload the conscious mind. Release of tension can be attained by expressive activities such as music and sports.

8.1.4 Disorder of addressing

Ideas (or delusions) of reference (IOR or DOR) take place when events in the environment are experienced spuriously as signals specifically directed towards the subject. The signal contents can be diverse, such as conversation, eye gaze, cough, noises in the environment, or messages in the television. In IOR the focus of the abnormality is not in the content of the information but in the 'address' attached to the information (which specifies who the signal is intended for). IOR is a phenomenon different from other delusions (although both can occur at the same time). IOR is better considered as a dimension within other delusional experiences. On its own it can be considered as a disorder of the 'communication address'.

The fact that such a phenomenon as IOR arises in psychopathology points to the existence of a healthy brain mechanism for 'address assignment'. When the address is not explicitly specified in the message, the recipient's brain is capable of automatically judging the address by the context and the content. Notably, this analysis is likely to have taken place before the content even fully reaches awareness. If the analysis is positive, the message is considered as self-related and conscious attention is then directed to the message. If the analysis is negative, the message is filtered from conscious awareness. The brain uses content of a message to judge pre-consciously whether the content should be further reviewed in consciousness.

When the filter is dysfunctional, spurious self-reference messages are identified. The mind interprets the messages as if they have already passed through the usual pre-conscious screening filter. This leads the mind to consciously attempt to extract significant meanings from the message, even though such meaning may not exist.

A 30-year-old gentleman expressed a belief that he has a chronic infection in his lungs, despite negative medical investigations. This symptom would normally be regarded as a 'hypochondriacal delusion'. He held this belief firmly on the grounds that in his presence people around him would soon start coughing. He interpreted this as evidence that micro-organisms from his infection were being transmitted to people nearby, resulting in their coughing. In this case, the primary anomaly appears to be the belief that coughing by the people around was related to himself, which led him to the secondary belief that he was the source of infection. In this perspective, the core feature of the delusion is 'reference' in nature. The 'infection' theme is a secondary elaboration to account for the reference experience.

8.2 Disorders of Agency

Information encountered in everyday life can be separated into the two streams of (1) semantic and (2) autobiographical information (Tulving, 1972). Autobiographical information may involve the possibility of personal action (or decision not to act). It is handled in a space that tracks prediction and outcome of actions. In contrast, semantic information is not linked to personal action.

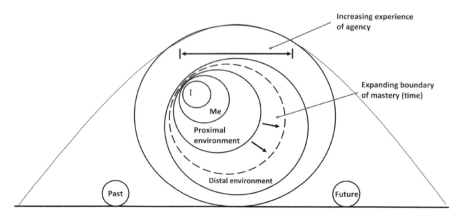

Figure 8.2. Semantic and autobiographical boundaries are defined by domains reachable/ controllable by one's actions. In the present, 'I' acts on 'me' and 'proximal' and 'distal' environments through social and physical contacts. The result is an expanding boundary of mastery, mediating an increasing experience of agency (see section 8.2).

Autobiographical information consists of learnt relationships between goal-directed actions and different types of outcome information that are potentially influenced by the actions. These relations are involved in the developing sense of 'self' in an early learning process where one learns that some aspects of the environment are within one's 'sphere of influence'. This 'field of control' is represented by aspects of the environment that share a higher probability of predictable change as a result of one's action. In this way a sense of agency (awareness of self-initiate acts) is central to the development of this 'sphere of influence' (see Figure 8.2).

8.2.1 Intentional representations of goal and agency

In a simple observation in the animal world, we considered how fishes swim in groups and maintain their relative positions with each other as well as keep steady their positions in relation to the seabed amidst changing sea currents. It is easy to see that 'internal representations' are involved, if not consciously, at least as a discrete unit in the motor computations for maintaining constant relative positions against perturbations (see Figure 8.3). In this example it is possible to view the 'goal' of 'maintaining a constant relative position' as a high-level goal. Computations that allow a perusal of the goal of keeping a constant position necessitate an integration of information about environmental perturbation as well as the current status and predicted action needed.

Having an internal 'goal representation' enables an organism to enjoy smooth execution of action and to cope with ongoing, superimposed, unpredictable environmental changes (just as factors such as wind, current, and terrain in locomotion).

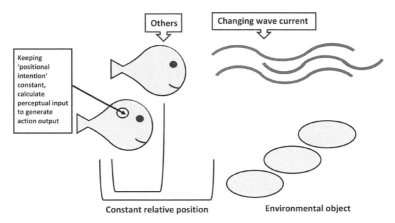

The fish maintains constant relative position, suggesting an internal representation

Figure 8.3. Internal goals and movements in a school of fish. Individual fishes are able to keep a constant relation position with other fishes and environmental objects. Movement is kept constant despite changing turbulence in the water. This suggests an internal representation to calculate perceptual input and motor output consistent with maintaining constant position in relation to the environment.

The fish, moving steadily despite water currents, calculates the additional resistance due to currents and acts to overcome the currents. The hummingbird balances itself in the air despite cross-winds. The computation involves some relatively invariant relationship with the environment that is monitored for action control. This relatively discrete, invariant cluster of information reflects an internal representation of the desired movement goal. The animal has to maintain a representation of some target state, which was set up prior to motion and then kept constant. It allows for comparison with the actual perceptual input in order to guide movement.

This monitoring of movement relative to goals and environment can be extended to human monitoring of the social environment. Jaspers (1913/1963) emphasized that the experience of reality has a 'quality of resistance', which must be overcome with intentional adjustments. This feature is consistent with the above account using a simpler example of animal locomotion. The awareness of resistance is an important aspect of the experience of reality.

Thus consideration of an intentional goal is important for an understanding of how the mind engages reality. The goal of homeostasis is to maintain a stable position in the social environment. Just as in motor monitoring, where the actual movements are compared to the goal and efforts are expanded to overcome resistance, the self with its social goals can also correct departures caused by perturbations. Active effort results in a sense of agency, and it is also instrumental in enriching a sense of self (see section 3.5).

Internal goal representations, even if not as a 'conscious' idea, are computed in order to guide actions and maintain position relative to environmental changes, such as sea currents. The goal-perception comparison is a basic feedback control system that creates contexts for actions. It gives rise to a sense of agency. If this system is not functioning, movement may be experienced as being controlled (alien hand syndrome, passivity) (Feinberg et al., 1992; Goldberg, 1985).

Disorders in agency result from failures of the mind to register intentional goal-directed actions initiated by the self. The symptoms of passivity and thought aliena-tion can be directly understood in this context (Frith & Done, 1989). The symptom of verbal hallucinations has also been related to a failure in internal monitoring of inner dialogues. The current framework unifies these accounts across the boundary imposed by conventional psychopathology (disorder of perception vs disorder of belief).

In disorders of agency the violation of a sense of 'predicted outcomes of actions' takes place in highly predictable relationships. They are usually experienced in one's own body (or that part of the body that is under voluntary control). However, in the modern technological world, they may extend to the proximal environment. For example, the sphere of predictable influence often extends to digital devices such as computers and mobile phones. The conventional boundary of the highly predictable spheres as defined by the biological human body is often extended to technological devices. The experience of unexpected outcomes in personal digital devices is indeed often encountered in contemporary psychopathology. A patient with psychotic disor-ders reports that their mobile phone does not react as predicted when they input com-mands, as evidence that some other agent is controlling their human-device system. The current conceptualization will enable this phenomenon to be understood as a passivity phenomenon extended to the persons' proximal environment. The mecha-nism of failed internal monitoring of the expected outcome of a self-initiated action is fundamentally the same as in previous conventional bodily passivity phenomena. This new way of grouping phenomena according to computational mechanisms may enable more informative studies of, for example, brain processes involved in psychopathology.

8.2.2 Disorders of inner dialogue

Inner speech is engaged to rehearse dialogue in encounters not only between self and others but also between representations of significant individuals in the inter-nal 'community of mind' (COM) representation (Hermans & Dimaggio, 2007). Representations of the 'others' emerge as a 'Bakhtinization' process (Bakhtinization involves a freeing of parameters to allow the representation to 'freely' evolve according to its own internal potential). While inner language can sometimes be used in more effortful problem solving, it can also be employed in a less explicit, more automatic process of inner expression in the COM. The Dialogical Self Theory proposed that within each individual's mind there are multiple representations of different people in their Lifeworld. These others' representations interact with each other through autonomous information exchanges. This exchange necessitates a large amount of information traffic in the brain between different identities, carrying messages that are propositional and linguistic in nature. The tagging of 'self-initiated' signals is an important marker for the 'self' as the source of these inner messages. If the tags are degraded, such inner information flow may be mistaken as externally generated verbal messages (hallucinations).

8.3 Disorders of Persons Representation

8.3.1 Disorders of information compartmentalization

Compartmentalization disorders involves the breakdown of 'source-information tagging' and results in the feelings of personal information being known widely.

Information in the mind is first distinguished between that which originates in one's own mind (self-generated) and that which one receives from another person (others-generated). Others-generated information is likely to be tagged according to its sources (Graesser et al., 1999; Senkfor & Van Petten, 1998). For self-generated information, there are tags about with whom this information has been shared (see section 8.2.2). The source and sharing status of a piece of information are important specifications of the information in a social context. This would have been important in an evolutionary stable (ESS, see section 2.4) prehistoric group environment because social information was valuable currency (see section 2.6). The value of a particular piece of information depends on its source and sharing status. When a piece of information is widely shared, its social market value reduces.

In the following treatment, notations are used for a clearer handling of the problem. Each piece of information $I1, I2, \ldots In$ held in the mind can be shared with a specific set of people (see Figure 8.4). The sharing tag (which we shall call information-shared tag IST) can be described as follows: $IST(0, A, B, C, all)$, where '0' is an empty set of 'no one', 'all' is the universal set of the entire population, 'A', 'B', and 'C' are particular sets of individuals, and 'S' denotes self. $I1[IST(0)]$ indicates that information 1 is shared by no-one else (i.e., a personal secret). $I2[IST(A)]$ indicates that $I2$ is shared by set A of individuals. $I3[IST(all)]$ indicates that $I3$ is openly shared by everyone in the reference group. In this way we can describe all the information in the mind by the general expression $In[IST(Xn)]$, n=1 to n, where n is the nth idea and Xn is the set of people sharing the idea In.

Interestingly, we note that this process defines another important parameter of the group as well. Individuals and their relationships can also be defined by their differential knowledge access. Each individual can be characterized by his knowledge profile (which ideas are shared with him). In this way we can express the sum total of knowledge for individuals and estimate the extent of their overlap (i.e., for A, B, C, etc. $Ia[IST(A)]$) (see Figure 8.4).

We can then consider the failure of information compartmentalization in psychosis: It involves an anomalous tag change in the IST value from '0' to '>0' for a significant amount of information. Ip[IST(0)] (Ip information was originally known only by self) becomes Ip[IST(>0)]. From the point of view of representation of individuals in A, B, C, etc. they are perceived by the self to be in possession of more information than they actually do in reality. This particularly concerns the previously Ip[IST(0)] 'private' information (note this is the information that is particularly poignant in terms of 'social calculus' and can be damaging to 'self' reputation and can lead to group rejection if shared). This model describes the perception that private information is being known by others in terms of representations.

After the formal description, we ponder on possible mechanisms for the collapse of differential tagging of information. It is prudent to estimate the communication pattern in the earliest evolutionary time scale: before human language fully developed, primordial communication was likely predominantly public, as gestural and simple verbal communication will be perceived by all people present in the surrounding, with little room for differential personalized information delivery; that is, there was only I(ISP all) or I(ISP 0).

It was only with the advent of written language that the possibility of selective private communication was enabled on a large scale; that is, S to A but not B was made possible.

The development of selective communication is highly significant, as it has enabled the use of information for group coalition. Information can be used to define in-group/ out-group status. It also creates the possibility for deception. This situation not only creates the need for tagging but also increasingly reinforces specific values for S-only information (i.e., self only). S-only information is 'personal secret'.

'S to A but not B' is made possible by 'addressing' (sealed information). The brain's cognitive module responsible for this function is likely to have evolved more recently and is demanding on cognitive resources. The 'S to A but not B' tag is important in social manipulation ('social calculus') because it generates the possibility for selective group bonding and deception. The ubiquitous presence of the seal in different cultures, from an early historical age, testifies to the importance of differential communication in human affairs. It also suggests that theory of mind (TOM) was developed initially for manipulation; that is, S wishes to manipulate others' TOM by controlling communication and uses S's representation of TOM (of A and B) to monitor this process. The differential tagging of 'S to A but not B' demands a high level of cognitive organization. This organization carries considerable resource implications. The more primitive situation of 'S to all' makes it more likely to be the default to settle back into when the cognitive capacity is compromised. When the interconnection between individual connections in the COM is strong, the collapse of the sharing tag may be sudden and follows catastrophe dynamics (see Figure 7.5 on catastrophe dynamics). This may provide an explanation for the pathological experience of 'thoughts being known by others'.

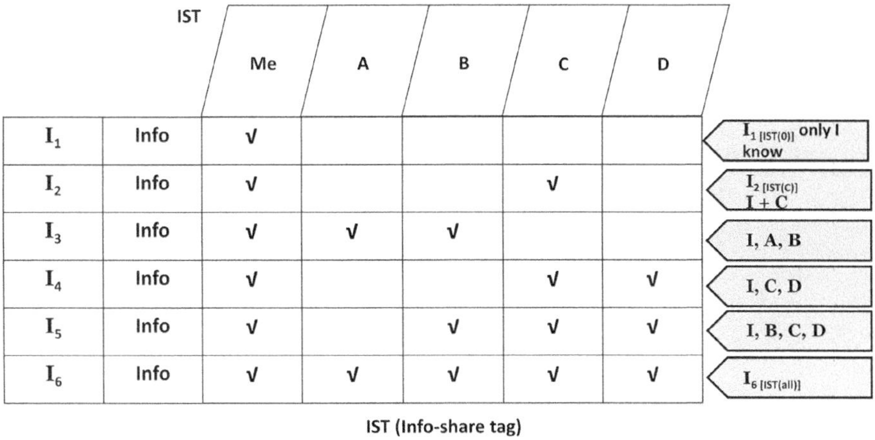

IST		Me	A	B	C	D	
I_1	Info	√					$I_{1\,[IST(0)]}$ only I know
I_2	Info	√			√		$I_{2\,[IST(C)]}$ I + C
I_3	Info	√	√	√			I, A, B
I_4	Info	√			√	√	I, C, D
I_5	Info	√		√	√	√	I, B, C, D
I_6	Info	√	√	√	√	√	$I_{6\,[IST(all)]}$

IST (Info-share tag)

Figure 8.4. Compartments of information. A, B, C, and D represent four other people. 'I1' to 'I6' are six pieces of information. Each piece of information is known by a specific set of individuals, summarized in the info-share tag from 'I1' to 'I6', ranging from 'only I know' to 'all'. Note that different sets of individuals are defined by the information sharing set (see section 8.3.1).

8.3.2 Disorders of automaticity

8.3.2.1 *Semi-autonomous representation of other people*

Importantly, 'other' representations are proposed here as 'Bakhtinized', semi-autonomous representations (see Figure 8.5 and section 8.2.2) (Lewis, 2002). For social predictions (TOM) to be effective, 'other' representations are allowed to operate in a way that is not tightly controlled by self-initiated directions (see Figure 8.5).

By design, 'other' representations operate using less directly controlled processes (see Figure 8.5) based on high-dimensional knowledge of other persons in the social world. The function of 'other' representations is to make predictions in the social world that can guide one's social behaviour. 'Other' representations are used for coming up with an estimation of 'what would I do if I were him?'; 'How would he feel if I were in his position?'; or 'what would he do, given what he knows?'. Most of these representations make use of social information encoded in a linguistic propositional structure. In real life, social information is often fuzzy and incomplete. As a result, heuristics and stereotypes are often used to fill gaps of information. This is open to biases and inaccurate predictions (e.g., stigmatization of mental illness is arguably a result of such processes). Proper handling of uncertainty is required (this may involve probabilistic reasoning and setting aside a costly space for alternative hypotheses to be retained for re-evaluation). The output of this social semantic estimation is largely held in a tentative-proposition linguistic structure.

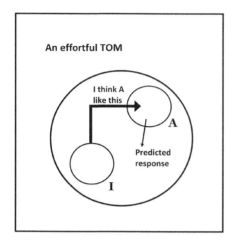 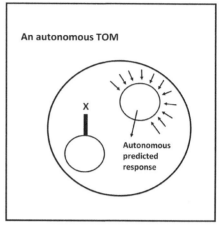

Figure 8.5. Autonomous TOM and COM. Left: an effortful TOM; in an effortful TOM 'I' makes deliberate estimation of A's response. Right: an autonomous TOM. In an autonomous TOM, 'I' refrains from making direct effortful estimations. Instead the response from A is allowed to settle by itself, taking into a wider range of information (see section 8.3.2).

The Dialogical Self Theory proposes that within the mind there are rich information exchanges between different representations of the self and others, using language-based representations (i.e., as in dialogues) (Hermans & Kempen, 1993). Applying the dialogical self approach, pathological phenomena relating to psychosis, autism, and personality disorders can be considered as consequences of malfunctions of TOM representations for significant others and the interactions between them. Failure of the TOM representations can affect subjective experience in a number of directions.

Failure to construct robust TOM results in a lack of TOM information to guide appropriate social behaviour (as in autism and Asperger's syndrome) (Baron-Cohen et al., 1985; Frith, 2004; Frith & Corcoran, 1996).

Failure to support probabilistic social evaluation may result in erroneous interpersonal interpretations. When the direction of bias is towards a direction that construes others as threatening, this results in paranoid tendencies and mis-attribution of hostile intention towards others (Green & Philips, 2004).

Inadequate information is particularly likely concerning others-to-others communication in the COM (see Figure 8.5). These links are not directly observable by the subject in real life. Indirect imputations have to be employed to evaluate these probabilistically (with high computational costs).

A dialogical approach can offer a potent explanation for verbal hallucinations. Verbal hallucinations may be viewed as 'runaway' inner conversational rehearsals that have lost their cognitive tags for internal self-initiation and are consequently attributed to having originated from the external environment.

In contrast to current theories of hallucination (such as the inner speech hypothesis, Jones & Fernyhough, 2007; McGuire et al., 1995, 1996), the current model is unique in offering a mechanism for explaining the phenomenological significance of third-person hallucinations as opposed to second-person hallucinations. Third-person hallucinations occur uniquely in the others-to-others space in the COM rather than in the others-self space. As 'others-self' dialogues are more commonly experienced (Lewis, 2002), corresponding hallucinations may emerge more easily with less extensive pathological processes. Others-to-others dialogues are less frequently experienced and require more extensive pathological processes to activate (hence the clinical significance of third-person hallucinations as a first rank symptom of schizophrenia, Schneider, 1959).

8.3.2.2 Spurious animation in objects

A young patient with autism spectrum disorder is very interested in primates. He has extensive knowledge on and intense interest in various species of primates. In a recent disturbance, he came across a stone statue of a particular primate species in

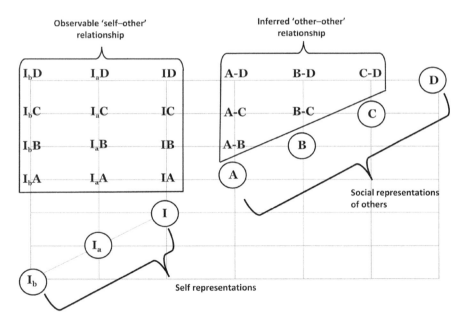

Figure 8.6. Self and Others representations. A, B, C, and D are 'Others representations' and 'Ib', 'Ia', and 'I' are self-representations, while 'IA', 'IB', 'IC', 'ID', 'IaA', 'IaB', 'IaC', 'IaD', 'IbA', 'IbB', 'IbC', and 'IbD' are observable 'self-other' relationships. A, B, C, and D are mental representations of other peoples, 'A-B', 'A-C', 'A-D', 'B-C', 'B-D', and 'C-D' are not directly observed by 'I' and has to be inferred as in 'other-other' relationships (see section 8.3.2.2).

a botanical and zoological park. He felt the primate statue communicated with him through telepathy and that the primate was pleading with him to bring it back to his habitat in Thailand. He experienced this communication with such strong conviction that he tried to remove the statue and was stopped by a security guard. In his representation of the primate statue, a notable individual variation is that he represents primates in a much more detailed taxonomy than others. He has been observed to be obsessed with animal toys. This is possibly a consequence of autistic tendencies leading to focus and emotional attachment to a narrow range of objects (primates) instead of people. The second notable feature is that his representation of the primate statue is animated. He attributed a TOM to the primate statue and experienced communication from the statue. This is despite the external object being a statue. The complex representation of a primate statue appears to be dominated by the activation of the 'primate' component and the neglect of the 'statue' component of the representation.

8.3.2.3 *Representations of self*

Owing to the cross-reference (mutuality) between semantic features, self-representations and 'other' representations can interact in rich ways in the semantic space. The evolution of self-representation is therefore closely associated with the status of representations of other peoples in the COM. Some aspects of the self are reflected in the representations of others. Each self-other relationship contributes to some aspects of the sense of self. The cumulative information serves to constitute an overall experience of self.

We shall try to describe this formally. The self (S) contains a number of self positions (S1, S2, etc.), each representing a subsidiary self in a particular role (self as a friend, self as a colleague, etc.). Other people (O) are represented by 'other' positions (O1, O2, etc.). Each of these representations Sn and On are constituted by a multi-dimensional vector of person attributes (this is fully articulated with the HICLAS model, Longenecker et al., 2016; see Figure 8.6). Formally, the relationship between these units can be accommodated with a matrix (S+O x S+O). Each element in the matrix is a link (relational links between objects) specified by one of several possibilities. In this matrix, various classic roles (archetypes) and narrative structures (cultural plots) can also be accommodated. The network is deployed by the mind to handle uncertainties in real life. There is uncertainty in most real-life social relations, particularly in O-O relationships to which S does not have direct access, except through gossips and through inferences.

8.3.2.4 *Failure of group synchronization*

In the mind of the individual there is a representation of the groups in their social environment (the COM). The individual interacts with the group and obtains information about the group. These items of information allow a comparison between the actual group and the representation of this group in the subject's mind. The comparison process will be compromised when there is a lack of contact with the actual group. It is also disrupted when top-down biases (see section 7.3) interfere with interpretation. The lack of information in the COM renders it vulnerable to top-down biases. A snowballing corruption of the COM can then result. Regular contact and information exchange are crucial to minimize the chances of a catastrophic corruption of the COM.

8.4 Disorders of Interactions between Representations

8.4.1 Disorders of context integration

In the human mind, top-down information allows complex behaviour to be adapted to and to be guided by previous experience. Dysfunction of top-down information flow results in specific abnormalities.

8.4.2 Top-down biases disorders

They involve the tendency of the mind to interpret ambiguous signals in a particular direction (e.g., self-blames or blaming others). The processing of information (constraint satisfaction) is biased by priming through partial activation of preferred patterns. Such priming may be influenced by a prevailing mood state or paranoid tendencies.

8.4.3 Confabulations

When the brain is compelled to respond while information is insufficient, it will compile a response based on the information available, even though the information may be grossly inadequate. In health, the individual has the capacity to refute the faulty response. In some conditions (such as neurological conditions affecting the function of the prefrontal cortex), the brain is not able to further evaluate the adequacy or otherwise of the compiled responses. Filling a focal information gap by default and failing to recognize the lack of information result in the clinical symptom of confabulation (Moscovitch, 1995). It is important to note that the natural tendency of the brain is to compose an 'understanding' based on whatever information at its disposal. The individual acquires in the course of cognitive development more advanced cognitive capacity to check this response. However, this later-acquired ability can be incapacitated in illness, resulting in the re-emergence of the primitive response to simply make sense from whatever material at hand. In a classic study of 'split-brain' subjects who had undergone commissurotomy (surgical division of the corpus callosum, which links the left and the right cerebral hemispheres), when the experimenter presented a funny cartoon in the left visual field of the subject, so that the image projected onto the right visual cortex, the subject laughed. He was then asked why he laughed. The questions and the response were processed in the left hemisphere, without the visual information of the cartoon. The left hemisphere constructed a response 'because you (the experimenter) look funny' with the information it has (facial muscle and auditory feedback confirming laughter, visual information of the experimenter), even though the experimenter did not look funny. This observation illustrates the tendency of the brain to make sense of available information by coming up with the best possible response, even though it may be inadequate.

A taxi driver in his 40s expressed the belief that he experienced tickling skin sensations in his head, which he could move at will around his body using Qigong. He believed that the sensations were caused by some micro-organisms, which he could move and eventually excrete. He examined his faeces and claimed that he could detect these organisms as 'worm-like'. When he was describing how he 'moved' the sensation (and the worms) in his body, he noticed a piece of towel on the desk, picked up the towel, and wiped his head in a certain direction. Then he said, 'I make use of the hydraulic forces in the towel, to force the sensation in this direction.' This is an example of a patient integrating incidental sensory information into an ongoing discourse. The process of gathering conveniently available information to weave into a response is confabulation.

8.4.4 The environmental dependency syndrome

Failure to use context results in over-relating to the immediate stimulus in constructing a behavioural response (see also section 8.1.2). This results in the environmental dependency syndrome. Examples of this syndrome are imitation behaviour and utilization behaviour (Lhermitte, 1986). In these conditions action is driven excessively by bottom-up information as a result of feeble top-down effects. In this situation, action can be initiated without a clear sense of agency (willed initiation). A 58-year-old gentleman with utilization behaviour was tested with a range of objects, spectacles, tendon hammer, and so forth, which he promptly picked up to use, regardless of how inappropriate the action was. When asked why, he could not respond clearly. After a while he said he just did it, as he is not sure whether it is a game. He could not elaborate further as to why he thought so (this is likely to be a retrospective confabulatory response).

8.5 Self-replicating Ideas in the Mind

The propagation of ideas in culture has been conceptualized as self-replicating units that observe rules of evolution. Principles for evolution of biological systems have been applied to the evolution of 'idea units', or 'memes', in culture (Blackmore, 1999; Dawkins, 1976; Humphrey, 1986). It has been argued that the same rules of biological evolution—replication, selective survival of the fittest (shaped by environments), and elimination by natural selection—can be applied to the realm of 'ideas'.

At the level of culture, the 'meme' theory has been applied to the propagation and survival of religious and political ideas in populations over time (Blackmore, 1999).

It is proposed here that some of the same approach can be applied to describe how ideas persist at the individual level, that is, reside *within* an individual. The survival of the meme at the individual level is different from the original consideration of meme dynamics at the population level. In culture, it is important to consider propagation *across* individuals using communication as the basic replication mechanism. In contrast, the persistence of the meme *within* the individual's mind involves selection and internal integration with existing semantic structures.

Why do some ideas but not others survive in a particular individual? This question can be addressed from both the properties of the ideas themselves and the properties of the host.

The 'adaptive' structure of self-replicating idea units (cognitive viruses) can explain why some ideas are more persistent than others. The host 'cognitive immunity' can also contribute to determine whether anomalous ideas are eliminated.

In one of the best-disseminated metaphors, the mind is likened to the soil upon which ideas grow. Some ideas grow, some are suppressed, and some are eliminated (Luke 8:4-15; Mark 4:1-20; Matthew 13:1-23, the Bible).

Ideas have to survive a 'semantic coherence screening' by the mind, depending on the extent to which they are in consonance with other ideas in the mind. We have already discussed how the meaning of ideas can be derived from the meaning of other ideas rather than purely from external reference (see section 6.1).

8.6 What Does It Mean for Ideas to Be Meaningful?

When incoming information arrives, an interaction occurs between the new information and the information existing in the mind. New information interacts with existing information to create updated representations.

New information relates to existing information in such a way that it constrains possible interpretations more than previously available information (otherwise it will not be new information). When the new idea arrives, not only does it carry new information but, collectively, a network of ideas linked to it acquires further information (see Figure 8.7). This new network of related ideas can be extensive. As they become re-organized in relation to other existing ideas, the global information level and coherence can be increased. Such information provides new latent possibilities for the entire network. The new idea brings forth some potential that has not existed previously. Therefore, the new idea contains information and new potentiality. This integration brings about a revision of high-level structures in the host (accommodation) (Piaget & Inhelder, 1969). The incoming idea and the existing idea interact in a way that generates new possibilities. It is important to point out that not all new ideas have this impact. Ideas too close to old ideas are redundant in that they do not contain adequate new information. Ideas too distant from the old ideas are too unrelated to be meaningfully integrated. A fruitful new idea has an optimal distance from the old idea. When

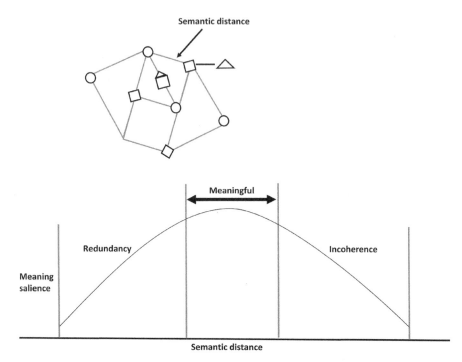

Figure 8.7. Semantic distance and optimal meaning levels. Top: semantic distance between a new semantic item and the existing semantic network that determines the extent to which the new item can meaningfully interact with the network. Bottom (from left to right): a schematic diagram depicting the inverted U-shape relationship between the level of meaning (salience) and semantic distance. When the distance is short, there is redundancy of information between the item and the existing network. When the distance is high, the item may not interact in a coherent manner with the existing network. At an optimal level of semantic distance, the new item brings significant new information to the existing network (see section 8.6).

integration occurs, we regard that idea as 'meaningful' as it imparts new information (Fauconnier & Turner, 2008).

In some pathological situations there may be difficulty in building up meaning. When ideas are redundant, they do not convey information (poverty of content of speech, Andreasen, 1979). When ideas are disconnected (loosening of association, Chaika, 1995), they also fail to convey meaning.

8.6.1 Clustering of mutually supporting ideas

Ideas cluster with related ideas to form coherent clusters. Compared with isolated ideas, ideas in a coherent group are much less vulnerable to being eliminated (see Figure 8.8).

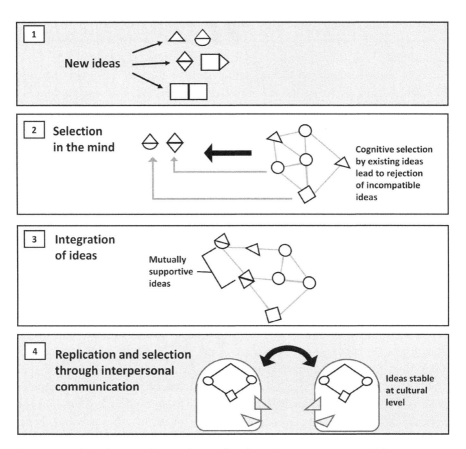

Figure 8.8. Self-replicating ideas in the mind and cognitive immunity. New ideas are generated in individual minds. Some ideas are rejected as being incompatible with the rest of the semantic system, while other ideas survive and persist in the individual mind. Ideas in an individual can be communicated to others and be rejected or supported. Through selection via interpersonal communication, ideas ascend from individual level to cultural level of existence (see section 8.6.1).

The notion that pathological symptoms may provide mutual support and reinforcement has been articulated in a 'symptom network' approach (Borsboom, 2017). A symptom network consists of a group of symptoms that may initially be triggered by an environmental event. The symptoms then act to cause intensification of other symptoms in the network and in this way reinforce one another. Eventually this may result in the persistent activation and stabilization of a network of self-perpetuating symptoms, even though the original triggering event may no longer be active. This approach has been offered to emphasize that symptom formation is not exclusively a result of direct biological brain anomalies, but the symptoms themselves (as subjective experiences) may *causally* induce the development and stabilization of other symptoms. The theory is a useful reminder that symptom formation may involve more than a simple unidirectional impact of brain events upon subjective experience. The theory however has some major shortcomings. It does not account for the delineation of symptoms: that is, what counts as one symptom. It is important to be able to delineate when two subjective events are regarded as two symptoms rather than one symptom. If symptom(s) exists in complex representations (as proposed in this account, see the treatment of dimensions in symptoms), it is not always clear how different components of a symptom might sometimes be considered as two separate symptoms. The co-occurrence of such symptoms is then not a matter of causality, but they are both instantiated by the same underlying complex mental representation. The current symptom network theory also falls short of providing mechanisms in which one symptom may be causally related to other symptoms. The representational approach proposed here is essential for understanding the delineation between symptoms and symptom complexes. Importantly, the representational account also suggests some potential mechanisms for causal interactions between symptoms.

8.6.2 Threatening ideas

The human brain has evolved to give more weight to potential risks and threats (Haselton et al., 2015). Ideas that contain elements of threats are difficult to dismiss in the mind. This phenomenon has already been discussed in connection with the survival of threatening themes in cultural memes (Grundlingh, 2017). Threatening ideas are particularly powerful when they are not open to being empirically tested. They are especially difficult to dislodge when they fit closely into the niches provided by narrative plots intrinsic to the mind. These features (threatening theme, not disprovable, contextual narrative coherence) can be powerful determinants of the survival of ideas of threats. Some threat-borne memes thrive particularly well in hosts with the risk-aversion proneness. These may account for contents commonly seen in psychosis (physical threats, threats to reputation) and in obsessions (fear of dirt, fear of forgetting).

8.7 Disorders of Offline Updating

Some computational updating of complex representations in the brain, such as the revision of stored schema, can apparently be carried out only while the system is not engaged with the environment. Such updating takes place when the system is offline (e.g., in sleep). Though not yet fully understood, this requirement appears to be a result of unavoidable hardware constraints in (at least) the vertebrae brain. Memory consolidation takes place in rapid eye movement (REM) sleep, which appears to be universal amongst all birds and land-based mammals. Representations appear to be incapable of being internally 'updated' simultaneously when they are linked to external perception and are 'in use'. As a result, offline dreaming is a necessary process for updating representations. If the system is prevented from offline updating there appears to be a limit beyond which computational failure may occur. It is well known that prolonged sleep deprivation can lead to psychotic experiences in healthy individuals (Frau et al., 2008; Petrovsky et al., 2014).

8.8 Disorder in Inter-individual Information Transfer

Language disorganization has been recognized as a phenomenon in the psychopathology of psychotic disorders (McKenna & Oh, 2005; Sims, 1995). It involves a situation in which linguistic communication from the subject is recognized by the recipient as 'disorganized'. It has been described as 'formal thought disorder' (disorder in the 'form of thinking') as disorganized speech is considered as evidence for disorganization in the underlying thought processes. Language disorganization is a unique phenomenon in psychopathology as it does not involve the subjective experience of the subject. In fact, the subject is often not aware of the communication problems and continues with the production of speech as if there is little awareness that the speech may not be understood by the recipient. The phenomenon is therefore located in the recipient of speech rather than the sender. Language disorder primarily involves the phenomenology of the recipient. It may be considered as an observation of the clinician involved in the dialogue. It is closer in nature to a 'clinical sign' than a 'symptom' (see section 1.1.2). Formal thought disorder has been described classically as deviations from a coherent 'stream of thought' (e.g., loosening of association, circumstantiality, tangential thinking, word salad). The current empathic representational account provides a comprehensive framework for understanding formal thought disorder.

Formal thought disorder involves transfer of information from the subject (sender) to the clinician (recipient). It often involves a dialogue process between the subject and the clinician. To provide a framework for formal thought disorder we consider information transfer (message) between the sender and the recipient. The information transfer is through language. The relevant information involves the content of intended communication in the sender. The process aims to convey this content to the recipient effectively, so that the information is represented in the recipient's mind. Formal thought disorder is detected when there is a failure in the transfer of information that cannot be accounted for by other processes (misunderstanding, failure in mechanical speech production, e.g., articulation, or general cognitive failure).

Failure in interpersonal information transfer can be considered from the perspective of information theory (see section 2.2). We can consider information transfer from the mental content of the sender (MSS) to the mental content of the recipient (MSR). Information is considered as the specification of one possibility amongst a range of possibilities. Information in MSS indicates that a specific content MSSi is specified amongst a range of possibilities MSSa, MSSb, MSSc, . . . During the language communication process, linguistic messages are communicated through a sequence of words that are uttered in a linear sentential structure (Wa, Wb, Wc, . . .). The sequence of words impacts on the mental content in the recipient MSR where it disambiguates the

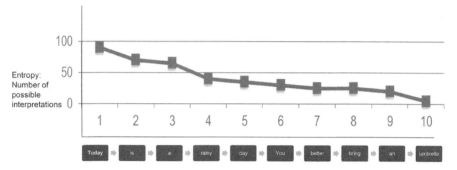

Figure 8.9. Schematic illustration of information transfer during verbal communication. Vertical axis: information, as expressed in the number of possible meanings at each stage of verbal communication. Horizontal axis: number of linguistic units verbalized. There is a reduction of the number of possible meanings as increasing number of units are uttered. The information carried in each unit can thus be conceptualized as the reduction in the number of possible meanings when that unit is uttered (disambiguation).

range of possible contents MSRa, MSRb, MSRc, ... to arrive at the intended MSRi. Let us analyse the relationship between Wa, Wb, Wc and the recipient mental content in more detail (see Figure 8.9).

Prior to the verbal communication, given the context, there are a range of possible contents for the recipient MSRa, MSRz, ... For example, let us say there are 100 different possible contents. The verbal message acts to specify which one out of the 100 possible content is the intended message. The sender uses words Wa, Wb, Wc to narrow down the possibilities. Each word uttered narrows down the possibilities to some extent. Since verbal communication is a sequential process (one word uttered at a time), information changes after each word W is received by the recipient. From the example of 100 possible MSR states, Wa narrows down the possibility to, say, 70. If Wa and Wb are meaningfully connected, Wb interacts with the remaining 70 possibilities and further narrows down the possibilities to, say, 50. If Wc is a less informative word (e.g., a frequently used, generic word) it may narrow the possibility only by a limited extent, say, from 50 to 40. Eventually, in a clear communication this process will lead to the possibility being narrowed to just one MSRi. The communicative process is then complete.

In formal thought disorder, there is a failure of this process, so that despite the use of an expected quantity of words, the possibilities in MSR fail to be narrowed down. A number of abnormalities may contribute to this failure. If Wa and Wb are not meaningfully related (i.e., the semantic distance between Wa and Wb is too large; see section 8.4.3), the arrival of Wb may not focus on the relevant subset of possibilities left after the initial specification by Wa. On the other hand, if the semantic distance between Wa and Wb is too small (i.e., if Wb is closely related to Wa), the information in Wb may be redundant, that is, similar to Wa so that it offers little independent contribution. The information conveyance of a particular word Wi depends not only on the one word W(i-1) preceding it but also on the other preceding words W(i-2), W(i-3), … The variation in semantic distance may be considered at different units spanning different numbers of words. For example, a two-word unit consists of Wa-Wb or Wb-Wc, while a three-word unit consists of Wa-Wb-Wc. If the decrease in semantic relevance occurs only at a larger unit (at the level of discourse), the resulting phenomenon may be a drifting direction in the discourse (the phenomenon of 'tangentiality'), with no loss of information that depends on the disambiguation from smaller units (i.e., word phrases or short sentences are meaningful). If the affected unit is smaller (at the level of several lexical items), the resulting phenomenon is a short sequence of words that do not make sense (the phenomenon of 'loosening of association'). If the basic grammar structure is lost (i.e., if Wa and Wb are also constrained by grammar), and this constraint is violated, the resulting phenomenon has been described as a 'word salad'. Failure of information transfer may also be a result of excessive use of generic words that convey little information (the phenomenon of 'poverty of content of speech'). Language disorganization is recognized both as a trait (persistent in patients regardless of whether in psychotic episode) and as a state (worsen in a psychotic episode). Disorganization is more severe when more abstract ideas are being communicated. There may be some content specificity in language disorder; that is, for the same subject, disorganization is more severe when certain content domains (often related to psychotic experience) are involved. It is not easy to parse out the effect of abstractness from content specificity.

Various cognitive theories have been forwarded to account for language disorganization in psychosis. They include theories of a generic cognitive (particularly attentional) failure and theories of disruption of the semantic system, that is, the structure of the semantic relationship between lexical items. A further possibility involves a failure of representation of the recipients' mental contents. Communication involves the intention to convey information from the sender to the recipient. For the sake of conciseness in messages (i.e., the Grice's maxim) the sender would be required to formulate the mental content (state of knowledge) of the recipient and to estimate the context as well as information that is already in existence in the recipient's mind. This 'linguistic' TOM in the sender is required for the formulation of the most efficient message to provide only the necessary information to the recipient. Under-estimation of the recipient's knowledge will result in the provision of unnecessary and redundant details (related to the phenomenon of 'circumstantial speech'). Over-estimation of the recipient's knowledge will result in inadequate information being provided for coherent understanding of the message. It may result in an increase in semantic distance between two words because the contextual link between them is missing, resulting in the phenomenon of 'loosening of association'. A young patient with psychosis was irritated when the clinician attempted to clarify the unclear references in his message and said, 'Why do you ask and pretend you did not know? You know I have communicated these to you already [through remote telepathy].'

8.9 Developmental Perspectives in Psychopathology

As a person develops, the structure and connections of the brain also unfold in a plan that is predetermined biologically, while the neural connections in the mind continue to deposit layers of unique individual life experience cumulatively over time.

The mind receives information from its experiential encounters in different life domains via cognitive 'structures'. Examples of these cognitive structures are body representation, self-representation, self proximal habitat representation, self-others representation, and distal external world representations (see Figure 6.8, Wernicke, 1881/2005). These representations are enabled in different stages of development. Pathologies can affect the brain and the mind during different stages. Earlier disorders may leave a broad vulnerability and set up a background for the impact of the later disorders. Developmental disorders (such as learning disability and autism) affect the earlier attainments of the developing mind; emergent youth-onset disorders (such as psychotic disorders and mood disorders) are likely to be unmasked by brain re-modelling processes during transition to adulthood. Degenerative disorders (such as dementia) impact on later life stages.

Developmental disorders are manifested from birth and are usually stable through-out the subsequent course of life. Early development sets limits to the global neural resource and computational capacity. If a representation is affected early, the effect is likely to be more devastating than when it occurs later, as it compromises upstream cas-cades, influencing a broad range of subsequent development processes. Developmental conditions such as learning disabilities, autism with TOM failure, and language failure (high-level language) can substantially compromise the unfolding potentialities in an individual. General intelligence has a particularly global role to play as it is involved in 'cognitive immunity' for ideas and resourcefulness in 'coping' with the messiness of life. It is a factor affecting the outcome of many mental health conditions.

8.9.1 Representational capacity in the developing brain

Homo sapiens have a relatively lengthy period of postnatal learning leading up to early adulthood. During this period, the brain accommodates a large amount of informa-tion. This includes basic acquisition of language and the subsequent elaboration of concepts, including social constructs and rules for relating to others. These cascades of developmental learning are plastic rather than hardwired, in contrast to inborn fixed action patterns in most animal behaviour (Lorenz, 1981). The preference of using adaptive learning rather than fixed wiring offers the advantage that they can accom-modate rapid changes in cultural contents. Flexible cultural learning is critical because the process can uniquely serve a vital function in defining social groups. Social group membership is confirmed by the sharing of cultural contents. Cultural contents change quickly through time so that individuals outside the group cannot infiltrate by super-ficial mimicry. Individuals are accepted in groups when they exhibit the possession of a shared cultural context. This necessitates a rapidly changing content that cannot be accommodated by biological hardwiring.

The semantic system matures as the inter-relationships between lexical units are enriched and consolidated. The semantic network becomes increasingly coherently connected (i.e., more 'mutuality') with growing cross-links between items. Through the rich, mutually supporting cross-links between shared units that map onto the external world, some of the hidden internal connections of the semantic network are expected to be consistent across individuals.

Around adolescence, the brain enters into a transitional developmental phase characterized by coordinated synaptic pruning, myelination, and maturation of inhibitory interneuron systems. These critical processes drive the brain's metamorphosis into an adult mode of operation. As an evolutionary adaptation, once adulthood is reached, the brain does not undergo further drastic modification to accommodate life experiences.

However, in the modern human life cycle, even after synaptic pruning is completed in the adolescent period, life experience often still has not yet reached saturation. The turbulent years of youth have extended further to an ever-lengthening period in modern communities (Arnett, 2000). This lengthy period is required for the acquisition of increasingly complex socio-cultural schemata. Increasing complexity of human society imposes growing demands on the brain's internal representations.

Originally the long maturation period of the human brain had probably evolved to adapt to the evolutionary needs for mastering language and social group structures. It is hard to determine whether it is possible to biologically further delay the closure of the brain's critical maturation period for an even longer period (Hensch, 2005). Even if it were possible, the pace of adaptation may not catch up with the pace of cultural changes eventually. Youths continue to be confronted with challenges of a mismatch between brain representational architecture and ever-increasing social-environmental processing demands. Originally the economy of the developing brain was designed to endow an organism with a high capacity for learning in childhood. The brain then becomes committed afterwards to adapt to the relatively stable natural adult environment in prehistoric hunter-gatherer ecology, that is, the evolutionary stable environment. The rapid evolution of the human environment in the last 10,000 years necessitated substantial adaptation, and this adaptation may not be fully attuned yet in the human brain (Harpending & Cochran, 2009). Accelerating changes in human culture and social organization have taken place only in the recent several thousand years. The need to cope with novel social structures in the late youth period where pruning has already been taking place may challenge the capacity limits for complex schemata. One potentially informative area of biological research is to investigate the mechanism for determining the window for brain plasticity and for pruning (Hensch, 2005).

The long postnatal period of brain growth and conceptual development in humans allows for a much richer interaction between the developing person and the environment. It also allows for more possibility of self-determination in which active choices and decisions may influence the developmental path (see section 4.2). In comparison, animal species with more maturely developed infants, although having a shorter period of dependence, allows less room for individualized paths in development. Genetics and brain hardwiring play a much greater role in determining the final behavioural patterns. In humans, the interplay between the unfolding of representational concepts, life experience, social interaction, and concepts of self allows the developmental path of the person to be determined by individual choice and culture as well (see sections 4.1.1 and 4.2).

In addition to the crucial events occurring in the brain in the youth period, external life experience is also expected to undergo quantal changes. In most societies, the individual becomes more independent as he departs from a childhood role and gradually takes on an adult role in the community. This involves forming relationships, belonging to groups, and establishing oneself in the community.

Many mental illnesses disrupt the actively evolving brain system during adolescence. Many major mental health disorders have onsets in late adolescence. The active brain synaptic modification in this period may be relevant to the onset of these disorders.

The brain synaptic pruning processes (e.g., by microglia) in late adolescence may be a key process in unveiling youth-onset mental disorders (such as psychosis and bipolar disorders). Pruning alters the computational properties of neural networks. Pruning of unused connections results in more specificity and efficiency, but the brain system also loses pluripotency and the capacity to compensate for dysfunctional components. This change can possibly expose latent inadequacy in underlying neural buffering capacity in vulnerable individuals and result in the decompensation of mental states (McGlashan & Hoffman, 2000). In a less adaptive neural network, there is less flexibility, more fixed-action patterns, more stereotypes, and more dependence on well-chosen initial connections. The less adaptive net will be less able to learn new patterns, and existing representations will be used for new situations even though they may not be optimal. New variations and refinements cannot be accommodated very well. Instead they are more likely to be ignored and only loose-fit matching will be available (see Figure 8.10).

The most important youth-onset disorders are psychosis (disrupting reality appreciation), bipolar disorders (disrupting dominance hierarchy behaviour regulation), mood disorders (disrupting negative bladder-space regulation), obsessive-compulsive disorder (disrupting negative bladder-space regulation), impulse control disorders, and addiction (disrupting self-control). It has been estimated that over three-fourths of mental disorders have an onset prior to 25 years of age.

In psychosis, there are a number of representational problems that involve how dopamine regulates higher social cognitive representations. The formation of mental representations of other peoples may be partly determined by early life experiences interacting with the current environment. Because of the changes in the modern human life cycle, high demands on adaptation are expected in the emerging adulthood period. There may thus be a mismatch between the timing of the biological neuronal pruning and the prolonged changes in complex social roles in modern societies.

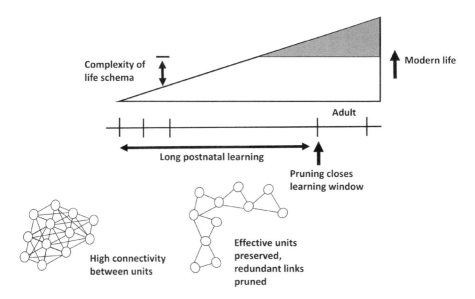

Figure 8.10. Pruning plasticity window and informational complexity with life course increased in modern life. Top: a long period of human postnatal learning leading to adulthood. Synaptic pruning closes the learning window at around adolescence times. Bottom (from left to right): In the pre-pruning network there is high connectivity between units, resulting in a plastic but less efficient system. Lower right: After synaptic pruning, effective connections are preserved and redundant links are pruned, resulting in more efficient and more specialized networks (see section 8.9.1).

After onset, the longitudinal course of psychosis depends on how the pathological representations dynamically interact with the remaining, healthy, representations. The course of a psychotic illness also depends on whether processes such as kindling are involved, as well as whether there is ongoing decline in neural resources. Using a representational approach will give fresh insight on the relationship between brain pathological processes and the courses of the disorders.

8.10 Summary

The approach currently proposed provides a novel framework for psychopathology. It focuses on mental representations as keys for understanding the relationship between the mind and the information it handles, as well as the problems that may arise when there are failures.

Mental representations provide a convergence between the phenomenological approach and cognitive models. Phenomenological work suggests the minimum composition of mental representation units involved in subjective experience. Parallel distributed models for these modules provide unique accounts converging with the phenomenological observations of psychopathological experiences. Key features of representations include a limited span of awareness and the use of generative linguistic structures to construct complex situational models to represent the social world. Mental representations handle information with constraints arising from the biological evolution of the human brain. This perspective enables the understanding of psychopathological processes as failures in information handling. Major groupings in psychopathological failures suggested by this approach differ from conventional categories in psychopathology in important ways.

A clear example is offered in the discussion on delusions. In conventional descriptive psychopathology, delusions are considered as 'disorders of content of thought'. Delusions are further classified according to their themes: for example, delusions of persecution, delusions of grandiosity, and delusions of reference. The current 'information-representational' account suggests a different framework that emphasizes the heterogeneity in the pathways towards 'delusions'. For example, instead of a unitary category of delusions, the current proposal suggests that delusions may arise from (1) top-down processing failures, (2) agency failures, (3) information compartmentalization, and (4) automaticity failures. In addition, from the mental representation perspective, the phenomena of delusions of reference are failures of 'addressing', not of 'contents'. They can thus be considered as a class of phenomena different from delusions. They are better considered as contributing one dimension to other forms of 'delusions'. The representational approach considers the evolutionary history of the human mind and suggests why psychopathological contents are not random but inherit tendencies that reflect the 'fault-lines' in the 'geology of the human mind' carved out from adaptations for early human survival. Through detailed analysis of representations of a social group, the current approach also provides a unique explanation for the significance of first rank schizophrenia symptoms, for example, third-person hallucinations and delusions of thought broadcasting. This new framework for psychopathology can generate new insights that enriches traditional accounts of mental symptoms.

9

Psychopathological Evaluation: The Clinical Dialogue

Evaluation in psychopathology takes place largely through a dialogue process in which the clinician negotiates access to anomalous experiences in the subject. The clinician also explores relevant background information about the contexts in which those experiences developed. In these processes, the clinician applies his empathic capacity in order to appreciate the contextualized experience of the subject (see Chapter 5 on empathy). We shall develop a framework for handling the clinical dialogue with more precision, using the concepts developed in this work.

9.1 Overview

The study of psychopathological symptoms as subjective experiences has been offered as a framework in phenomenology (see section 1.2.1). Phenomenology emphasizes a disciplined assessment of subjective phenomena, in particular the 'suspension of judgment in the process of attending to and extracting primary experiences' (Husserl, 1913, 1921/1970, 1913/1931, 1936/1954; Jaspers, 1913/1963). It is recognized that a tendency in human thinking is to simultaneously grasp the primary experience and generate secondary interpretations. It is important for the clinician to segregate secondary interpretations from primary experiences in the process of describing subjective phenomena. Phenomenology aims at a minimalist approach. It starts with the most parsimonious basic components of subjective experiences (see Chapter 3). The approach is thus relatively free from the theories of different schools of psychology. The basic components of experience as clarified in phenomenology can later be utilized by a variety of psychological, psychotherapeutic, and neurocognitive theories downstream. However, for psychopathological evaluation, the objective is to stay as close as possible to the primary phenomena.

It may be counterintuitive to appreciate that it requires more effort to stay free from theoretical involvement. This point can be illustrated using the historical evolution of pottery craft in ancient China as a metaphor. In the evolution of the glaze (decorative coating) in ceramics, the first glaze to emerge was not the colourless or white glaze but the green glaze (made from selected ingredients from the soil), which was developed around AD 100. It took another 400–500 years before the white (or transparent) glaze was developed in the sixth century (the 'white' glaze is actually transparent, applied over a white body). In psychopathology as well as in ceramics, the technique of a colourless cover layer requires more techniques and distillations. The information we can then attain may enjoy closer proximity to the core pathological processes and enable us to achieve better prediction of illness trajectories.

The clinical dialogue is an evaluative technique in psychopathology involving an iterative process (Pickering & Garrod, 2004). Through cycles of information exchange between the patient and the clinician, the psychopathological experience is progressively clarified. The clinician has the opportunity of probing for information as the model is being developed. A well-managed clinical dialogue involves many different skills.

The overall objectives of the clinical dialogue are threefold.

(1) A psychopathological 'clarification'. The 'psychopathological clarification' involves detailed clarification of anomalous experiences in terms of their representational structure and content. This includes the primary experience, the contexts, and the development path of the anomalous experiences. The clinician also observes the patient's behaviour, including how he engage with the clinical dialogue itself, as well as other signs of observable behavioural abnormalities.

(2) A detailed perspective about the patient as an evolving Person, developing through a chosen path of engagement in his Lifeworld. The anomalous experience is placed in the context of the Person by considering the basic structure of the Person and the representations in his Lifeworld.

(3) Optimal engagement of the patient so that future therapeutic interaction will be facilitated (Shea, 1998).

9.2 Preparations for Clinical Dialogues

9.2.1 Engagement

Engaging the patient and building up a working rapport are not trivial processes in mental health consultations. While in general medicine patients are driven to seek help to relieve distress, in mental health clinical scenarios this drive is often lacking. Patients with mental health conditions often have limited appreciation of their problems (Marková, 2005; Tait et al., 2003). Patients tend to seek help reluctantly and disengage easily, aggravated by heavy stigmatization. Clinicians have to deploy extra effort just to engage patients. The process of engagement starts from the very first contact. Often, the initial evaluation is also the beginning of a therapeutic relationship. Sufficient attention to the interactional processes is crucial to the efficient conduct of assessment and to facilitate future therapeutic work with the patient (Shea, 1998).

9.2.2 Clinical etiquette

An evaluative interview is a unique encounter between two individuals. Within the approximately one-hour interview, the clinician aims to gather high-quality information that allows an accurate clarification of the anomalous experiences. This is a challenging task in view of the limited time frame.

A respectful introduction, stating the location, the time and the context of the interview, is a good start to a professional encounter. Defining a professional encounter explicitly is important as it evokes a professional-client schema rather than the schema of an informal encounter between friends. The professionalism enables explorations in areas that are inaccessible in informal friendly interactions. However, having defined this context, it is then desirable to generate an atmosphere that still enjoys the ambience of a friendly sharing.

9.2.3 Information quality

Clinicians should be mindful of potential sources of 'noise' in psychopathological information, as they may compromise clinical decisions. The quality of the clinical dialogue depends on the processes of the interaction as well as the individual characteristics of the clinician and the patient.

The contents covered by a psychopathological interview comprise subjective experiences of the patient. Access to subjective experiences is negotiated through a skilfully conducted dialogue. Factors such as language and differences in interpretation may constrain how the experience is communicated and received (see section 9.3 on the dialogue cycle). While it is important to recognize some limitations in access to subjective data through dialogue, it is equally important to be aware that with due attention it is possible to clarify high-quality data concerning subjective experiences (see section 9.2.4).

The approach currently proposed involves considering subjective experiences as structured phenomena. They can be described as mental representations consisting of feature dimensions (see Chapter 6). Clarifying a subjective phenomenon involves identifying which dimensions are involved as well as what contents fill the dimensions. It is also important to identify the contexts in which the anomalous experience took place.

'Thick description' is a method that involves making explicit the details about the experiential contents and the contexts. In a summary account, inevitably some data are filtered out at an early stage, thereby increasing the possibility of undiscovered bias in the selection of data. When raw data are richly represented, the context under which specific information emerged becomes available for subsequent examination. Without detailed information about the context of the observation, it becomes more difficult to evaluate, especially when apparently contradictory information arises at different points in the interview process.

An experienced clinician does not regard contradictory information with the assumption that there must be some 'error' and only one of the accounts can be 'correct'. Discrepancies can be genuine and informative, if the contexts in which different observations are made can be explored. This may lead to a more informed grasp of the patient's experiences. Clinical notes in psychiatry should be rich and sufficiently detailed, rather than being merely a checklist.

9.2.4 'Immersion' in the patient's Lifeworld

In a psychopathological interview, an interviewer aims to gain access to the psychopathological phenomena that take place in the subject's daily life. In order to do so competently, it is important that the interviewer has an adequate grasp of the Lifeworld of the subject (see section 1.2.1). While there are limits to the extent to which the interviewer can directly observe the subject experiencing his world in a real-life situation, it is important for clinicians to have extensive contact with the socio-cultural environment in which the subject lives. The meaning of the experiences can be accessed in this context through the use of empathy (Geertz, 1973). Adequate socio-cultural contextual exposure for the clinician is crucial for understanding a patient's experiences. The task of the clinician is to connect to the subject's world and to empathize how this world is experienced by the subject. The access to meaning is possible via the interviewer's own subjective experience of the world and meaning system. This way of understanding is described as 'verstehen' by Jasper (1913/1963) and has been elaborated by ethnographers in anthropology. Indeed, the psychopathologist has to become 'immersed' in the observation process. Through this immersion, his own system of meaning and Lifeworld of the subject will then become tools in understanding the subject's experiences.

9.2.5 Active probing and 'clinician participation effects'

One of the factors that affect emerging information in a clinical dialogue is the impact of the interviewer. The interviewer's behaviour affects the emergence of subjective data. It is important to recognize how much of this data is influenced by the interviewer's style and how much is the result of the primary experience of the subject.

In a psychopathology evaluation, the interviewer is not just a passive observer but an active participant in a process of dialogue in which psychopathological experiences are clarified. It is important for clinicians to be mindful that they have an impact on the phenomena under observation (Oswald et al., 2014; Robins et al., 1996).

This situation, where the observation process impacts on the observed phenomena, is often encountered in scientific studies. For example, crystallography is an important technique in the observation of protein structures. Protein 'crystals' are analysed using x-ray. The crystallization, however, extracts protein from its natural environment, which is a fluid medium. Different domains of science devise their own methods to tackle these kinds of problems. In the study of psychopathological phenomena, this involves a disciplined attempt to dissect the various additional embedded layers of information resulting from the observation processes.

When the interviewer is aware of the dual-role of being an observer and a participant, these two roles can be complementary rather than compromising each other. The observer actually can make a more in-depth observation through the use of active exploration processes. This approach has been discussed earlier (see section 5.1.2 on empathic explication).

Is it possible to 'distil' the primary subjective experience from the product of interactional processes? Some insight can be obtained by repeatedly approaching the same experience through different perspectives. When the same content is approached from different angles, the resultant dialogues have overlapping and non-overlapping contents. The interviewer can tease out how much consistency there is in the core expression and how much variations are dependent on the different conversational contexts. In a previous discussion (see section 6.5.1), we have seen how the previous states of mind (SOMs) affect the current SOM. If we attempt to address the current SOM from a number of different pathways (i.e., each time through a different SOM pathway), it may be possible to compare the different SOMs we obtain and extract the core that is consistent. This exploration is similar to the manual exploration of an object by touch from different angles (see section 5.1.2 on empathic explication).

Adequate probing is mandatory for unveiling complex subjective phenomena. Probing refers to the process in which the interviewer actively interacts with the subject in an attempt to facilitate the description of the phenomena. This requires the subject to actively retrieve and explore his own inner experiences in ways beyond what he has offered in the first place. Active probing offers a good opportunity to observe how the patient comes up with responses. Situations in which the subject has to give a forced-choice response are considered more vulnerable to the tendency of *ad hoc* response instead of genuine reflection of inner experiences.

A single phenomenon can be probed from different angles using different lines of approach. This may yield different results. Having a grasp of the different descriptions that emerge from different probes enables a more in-depth appreciation of the phenomena under observation (see section 5.1.2 on empathic explication).

It is also important to consider whether the subject has reasons to intentionally conceal information or to mislead the interviewer. It is acknowledged that deception and concealment can take place in clinical interviews. Intentional deception may be difficult to unveil, and it would take time and effort to detect inconsistency that is attributable to deception. There is no substitute for adequate probing. Deception and concealment, apart from leading to a distortion of the information, can themselves be significant signals in psychopathology.

9.2.6 Behavioural observations

At the same time that clinician immerses himself in the clinical dialogue, he also takes up the role of an observer on a patient's verbal and non-verbal behaviour, including the ongoing interactional dialogue processes in the interview. Though the observation takes place during the clinical dialogue, the information obtained in this way includes clinical signs (rather than subjective accounts) that fall under the premise of the Natural Sciences (see section 1.1.1). One example is the observation of the patient's speech in order to decide whether language disorganization occurs. Language disorganization is an important clinical sign. Pragmatic procedures to observe and identify language disorganization have been detailed (e.g., Chen et al., 1996).

It is important to recognize that attention to context is also important in behavioural observations. For example, language disorganization is more observable in some content areas than in others (e.g., when discussing more abstract topics or topics related to the content of psychotic experiences).

9.2.7 Perspective switching

One of the basic skills for clinicians involves a switching among three perspectives: a first-person perspective, the patient's perspective, and a third-person perspective on the part of the interviewer. In the first-person perspective, the interviewer is fully engaged in the interview process as a participant in a conversation. Therefore, the immediate experience of the interviewer is as a person experiencing a conversational process with the subject. In empathic understanding the clinician tries to see things from the patient's point of view. In addition, the clinician 'literally' scans the visual environment from the subject's perceptual viewpoint (see section 9.6.1.4 on visual environment). On other occasions, the interviewer switches to a 'third-person perspective' from time to time (Libby et al., 2009). In the third-person perspective, the interviewer inspects the interview process as if through the eyes of someone observing the interview from the outside. This third-person perspective enables the interviewer to reflect on the interactional processes taking place between himself and the subject. Intentional and regular switching between these perspectives is a skill the clinician develops with practice.

9.3 The Clinical Dialogue Cycle

The clinical dialogue involves a transfer of experiential information from the patient's mind to the clinician. The aim of the clinical dialogue is to build as accurate as possible a representation of the patient's psychopathological experience as a mental model (representation) in the clinician's mind. A visualization of the steps involved in the dialogue cycle is a tool that clinicians can utilize during real-time monitoring of the interview process (see Figure 9.1).

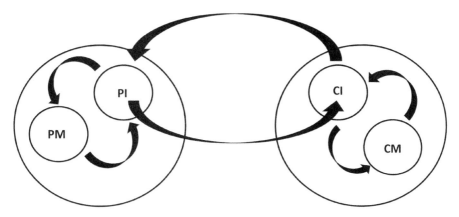

Figure 9.1. The dialogue cycle. The transfer of information from the representation in the patient's mind to the clinician. PM: part of the patient's mind experiencing the psychopathology; PI: part of the patient's mind involved in communication with the clinician; CI: part of the clinician's mind involved in communication with the patient; CM: part of the clinician's mind allocated to building a model of PM (see section 9.3).

9.3.1 Components of the clinical dialogue cycle

There are four basic modules involved in the dialogue cycle, consisting of an experience module (M) and a communication module (I) for both the clinician (C) and the patient (P). Within the clinician there are two modules. One module (CM) is set aside for constructing a representation of the patient's symptoms. Another module (CI) is responsible for communication with the patient. Similarly, in the patient's mind there are two modules. One module (PM) is where the patient experiences psychopathology. The other module (PI) is involved in communication with the clinician. These modules are related to one another as described in the basic structure of the 'atomic representation of experience' (see Figure 9.1).

The communication modules in the patient and the clinician are engaged in iterative cycles of conversation. If the communication module in the patient is itself directly affected by illness (such as via language disorganization), the dialogue cycle can be significantly compromised.

9.3.2 Processes in the dialogue cycle

9.3.2.1 *Process 1: Initiation of the clinical dialogue cycle*

The dialogue cycle starts when the patient begins to give an account of the symptoms that he has been experiencing. The clinician aims not to constrain the dialogue. The patient is allowed freedom to choose how to approach the area or experience that concerns him most.

9.3.2.2 *Process 2: Patient accesses his own experience*

The patient refers to the part of his mind where the anomalous experience took place (his experience module). This process of self-observation on the patient's part assumes that the patient can relate to his experience as an observer from one part of his mind that could make observations on another part of his mind (see section 3.4.2). Sometimes, the phenomenon being observed is in the past and memory processes are involved (see section 3.4.3). When the target processes accessed are in the present, a self-reflective process is implicated. These processes enable the grasping of an internal experience that can then be communicated. The phenomenon that is grasped can be specified with the structure of a representation, with dimensions that can be filled. It should be noted that the capacity for reflection may not always be entirely intact. It could be impaired, for instance, during an acute psychotic state. In psychosis, the cognitive space for reflective processes may be compromised by the immediacy of the psychotic phenomena.

9.3.2.3 *Process 3: Patients communicates their experience*

The success of communication depends on the integrity of a number of factors. First, the communication module in the patient has to be competent and willing to engage. Second, the patient has to be able to encode the relevant experience in terms of linguistic expressions available in his language.

To the extent that the semantic network is culturally shared between different individuals, experiential states could potentially be communicated between individuals. Experiential information is transferred to linguistic expressions. It is important to understand that linguistic representation of experience is a processed representation of the experiences rather than the raw experience itself. Proper communication of experience depends on the richness of the subject's linguistic resources as well as the availability of relevant vocabulary within the shared language itself. For instance, it is well known that different languages vary in their richness for descriptors of emotions (Russell, 1991).

9.3.2.4 *Process 4: Clinician receives the communication*

When the clinician receives verbal utterances communicated by the patient, he decodes the patient's messages and uses the information to construct a model of the patient's experience. The clinician allocates a cognitive space in his own mind for building up a mental representation with the data communicated by the patient. However, the information needed for building up the representation may be incomplete. In the absence of specific information, the clinician may utilize contextual information to fill the gaps. It is important for the clinician to be aware of such processes in his own mind. Excessive 'top-down' filling in of gaps may overshadow 'bottom-up' information from the patient. In this situation the stereotypic expectations of the clinician may override the primary experiential details provided by the patients. Such biases can lead to a model that does not accurately reflect the patient's experience.

Complex processes take place in the clinician's mind to evaluate the model that is being built up. This reflective process involves the ability to distinguish between internally anticipated information and externally received information (a form of source memory for the clinician). The reflection will distinguish what is already known from what is still not yet ascertained. The ability of the clinician to evaluate the emerging model is extremely important in guiding the clinician himself to generate further questions in the dialogue cycle.

9.3.2.5 *Process 5: Clinician constructs model of the patient's experience*

The psychopathological experience is initially private to the patient (see section 5.2.3 on the limits of empathy). The clinician can access the information only through the process of an empathic dialogue, using linguistic concepts inherited in a shared culture as a tool for clarifying the psychopathological experience. With these caveats, a limited but valid model of a patient's experience can be constructed.

We note that the representational structure of the psychopathological experience in the clinician's model may not be the same as the representational structure of the primary experience in the patient. The representation of primary experience is embedded in layers of further processing (see Figure 9.2). The clinician may have to use information from these additional layers to disambiguate and reverse-estimate information in the primary representation. Various active probing possibilities can be deployed to further clarify the primary experience in a process of explication.

Clinicians can also be vulnerable to premature closure in the model construction process, when excessive top-down information is employed in the clinician's mind to 'fill in' what the patient has not communicated. To minimize these tendencies, attention to the phenomenological practice of 'suspension of judgment' is a particularly essential skill for the clinician. The ability to keep close to the primary experiences of patients is important for the validity of the psychopathological observations. In developing a model for the patient's psychopathological experience through clinical dialogue, the congruence between the patient's and the clinician's linguistic representations will affect the extent to which an accurate model can be effected. Therefore skilful linguistic alignment in the clinical dialogue is also an important prerequisite.

9.3.2.6 *Process 6: Evaluation of the model leading to new exploration in the next iteration*

In the process of constructing the model of the psychopathological experience, the clinician seeks the most efficient approach to the next cycle in order to obtain discerning information that can help discriminate between the different possibilities in the remaining part of the model. From an information perspective, a partially filled model still contains parts in which several possible options remain viable. Further information is required to distinguish between these options (see section 9.2.3 on information). Gaining information for this purpose requires clinicians to anticipate the kind of questioning that will lead to the most discriminating information. Ineffective questioning will generate responses that do not adequately distinguish between the remaining possibilities.

The processes of acquiring information that take place in a clinician's mind can be illustrated by the 'animal guessing game'. In the game, the host identifies a target animal in his own mind, say 'elephant', but does not disclose this to the participant. The participant has to guess what the animal is by asking questions that the host has to answer truthfully. Examples of questions are 'Does it have fur?' and 'Can it fly?'. The participant aims to arrive at the correct animal in the shortest possible time. Let us consider a step in the middle of the game where the participant already has some information about that animal. His task is to generate the next question such that the response to that question will carry maximal information. From the information perspective, the game involves starting with the whole set of 'all animals' at baseline (low information). Each question and response generates information by eliminating some possibilities. For example, 'lives on land' will remove sea animals and narrow down the remaining number of possibilities. A statement that specifies only a few possibilities will be highly informative if confirmed. However, their chances of being confirmed are also smaller. The use of such a question approximates random 'guessing'. The converse is also true: The asking of a condition that contains a large number of possibilities (e.g., does it have legs) is likely to be answered affirmatively but does not narrow down possibilities in a powerful way. Some questions will be redundant if they do not narrow down further possibilities effectively. Ideal questions should reduce the possibilities, approximately by half. In this case 'luck' is involved to a lesser extent, no matter whether guessing was correct or not and the remaining possibilities are reduced. The clinician in a clinical dialogue has a similar task. What is the question that would be the most effective in extracting maximum information such that more alternatives are ruled out? Generating this question requires considerable knowledge about the universe of anomalous mental experiences.

9.3.2.7 *Clinician's reflection on the clinical dialogue*

During the clinical dialogue, an experienced clinician can often judge reflectively the quality of the model being constructed. When difficulty is experienced, the clinician will be aware that he is not achieving an adequate clarification of the patient's symptoms. On this occasion, it may be helpful to identify the source of the limitation by reviewing the steps involved in the iterative clinical dialogue (see Figure 9.1). The clinical dialogue cycle is designed as a pragmatic tool to facilitate such a review, even in real time during the interview. Obstacles can arise in any of the steps of information transfer highlighted in this model. Smooth information flow in all steps contributes to the quality of the final model.

9.3.2.8 *A model of the clinical dialogue*

A model of the clinical dialogue is presented using ideas that have been developed in the previous sections (see Figure 9.1). The model incorporates the use of representations in the patient's and the clinician's mind and attempts to describe the process of transfer of psychopathology information between the different components.

The key components of the model are described here. In the patients there are two compartments, the 'I' that is communicating with the clinician (PI) and the 'me' that experiences the potential psychopathology (PM). In the clinician, there is the 'I' that communicates with the patient (CI) and the part in the clinician that is assigned for phenomenological understanding of the patient's 'anomalous experience' (CM). The aim of the clinical dialogue process is to extract as much information as possible, and as accurately as possible, from the patient's 'anomalous experience' (PM), to be represented in the clinician's model (CM). CI and PI are involved in the explicit clinical dialogue for this purpose. PI and PM as well as CI and CM are involved in internal information exchanges. We use a constraint satisfaction process in a parallel representation to denote the content in each of the PM, PI, CI, and CM components. The constraint satisfaction process allows pattern completion from memory. The goal of the clinical dialogue is then to generate in CM a model that approximates the informational

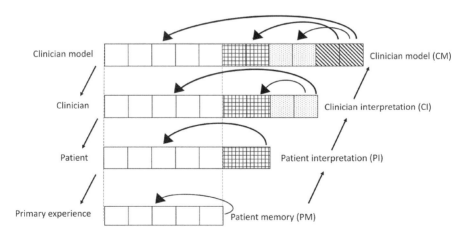

Figure 9.2. Embedded information layers in the clinical dialogue. Bottom to top: primary experience in patient memory (PM), patient's interpretation (PI) of the primary experience, clinician's interpretation (CI) of the patient's communication, and clinician model of the patient's experience (CM) (see section 9.3.2).

content of PM as far as possible. Yet, CM does not have direct access to PM, and explicit information transfer can only take place via PI and CI.

Suppose PM contains a representation for a subjective phenomenon (e.g., an auditory hallucinatory experience). The structure of the PM representation contains a number of dimensions relevant to an auditory hallucination (e.g., intensity, frequency, acoustic clarity, control, semantic content, number and identities of interlocutors, second or third person, spatial information, and emotional response). The patient's experience of hallucination fills these dimensions by specifying each dimension. It is possible that some experiences are less well formed and fill only some of the dimensions (i.e., sometimes *dimensions* might be missing, e.g., spatial information or personal identity information). In these situations, identification of the missing dimensions in the representation is just as important, as it contributes towards characterizing the structure of the representation (i.e., some specific dimensions are not represented). Previous studies have suggested that some feature dimensions of hallucination may map to brain states (e.g., spatial locations) and may have diagnostic and prognostic significance. It is important to appreciate that when primary experience took place in $PM(t0)$ (say, 24 hours ago), top-down and bottom-up processing may have already occurred. Subsequent to the primary experience, memory consolidation processes may also have taken place (e.g., incorporation of secondary ideas to make sense of the hallucinatory experience). These layers of initial processes have already ensheathed the primary experience before it is further accessed in $PM(t1)$. It is important to recognize that unlike $PM(t0)$, which is a primordial experience, $PM(t1)$ is a memory representation. $PM(t1)$ may contain more dimensions than $PM(t0)$. In addition, some unfilled dimensions in $PM(t0)$ may be filled in $PM(t1)$. Thus $PM(t1) = PM(t0) + PMc(t1)$, where PMc denotes memory consolidation in PM.

In response to the communication with the clinician (CI), the $PI(t1)$ component of the patient accesses the $PM(t1)$ representation in search of information in specific dimensions. This is carried out iteratively over individual dimensions one at a time. That is, CI may explicitly request PI to inquire about one feature 'n' in $PM(t1)$. After feature 'n' is clarified, CI may enquire about the next feature, 'n+1'. This process is repeated until CI is satisfied with the model being built in $CM(t1)$. The CM space is initially blank, and incoming information from PI via CI is used to specify dimensions in $CM(t1)$. In the communication between PI and CI, linguistic symbols are aligned such that information can be conveyed as accurately as possible (e.g., a word used by PI should map onto similar meaning in CI). However, in the information transfer from PI to CI, PI tries to make sense of $PM(t1)$, and this process may add information to $PM(t+1)$ in order to match constraints consistent with PI interpretation of PM. We can express this component as $PIu(t1)$ (PI's unique contribution to $PI(t1)$). Thus $PI(t1) = PM(t1) + PIu(t1)$. If we consider further processes leading to $PM(t1)$, that is, $PM(t1) = PM(t0) + PMc(t1)$, we have the following relationships:

$$PI(t1) = PM(t1) + PIu(t1)$$
$$PM(t1) = PM(t0) + PMc(t1)$$
$$PI(t1) = PM(t0) + PMc(t1) + PIu(t1)$$

In other words, the patient's awareness of psychopathology is a result of the primary experience, memory consolidation, and alignments with his own subjective viewpoints.

This information is what is conveyed to the clinician at $CI(t1)$. When the clinician receives the information, the information is interpreted within a context of the clinical dialogue, and depending on the level of alignment, the clinician may fill the information to some extent with his own ideas as a result of communication gaps (e.g., what the clinician and the patient understand by 'just before sleep' may be different).

Likewise, when the clinician places the information in CM, existing contents may affect the interpretation of the arriving contents. Such priming is exacerbated by a closed and inflexible mindset. An open, reflective, empathic attitude in the clinician may reduce such biases in the CM component.

Thus the information that is finally communicated to the clinician is

$$CM(t1) = PM(t0) + PMc(t1) + PIu(t1) + CIu(t1) + CM(t0)$$

$CM(t1)$ is the actual information that is available. From $CM(t1)$, the clinician intends to access $PM(t0)$ as much as possible. The task for the clinician is then to have some estimation of the other components $PMc(t1) + PIu(t1) + CIu(t1) + CM(t0)$. If more information about each component is available, these might be used to estimate the extent of their contribution to $CM(t1)$. By subtracting these from $CM(t1)$, we can potentially enhance the information about the original $PM(t0)$ representation.

$$PM(t0) = CM(t1) - (PMc(t1) + PIu(t1) + CIu(t1) + CM(t0))$$

$CIu(t1) + CM(t0)$ are accessible to the clinician. With training and reflective practice, the clinician can learn to be more aware of these components. In estimating PMc and PIu, the clinician often has to retain a broad range of information about the context of the communication in order to have more ideas about the contributions of Plu. It is therefore important that the clinician, in the process of communication, takes in the wider dialogue context as he deploys his empathy towards grasping the primary experience in the patient. The grasp is necessarily complex and not primordial. What is aimed at is information about $PM(t0)$ that is embedded in $PI(t1)$. As the clinical dialogue unfolds, the clinician has the opportunity to actively probe for information in an explication process. The probe can be about $PM(t1)$ or one of the sub-components therein (e.g., $PMc(t1)$ or $PIu(t1)$). For instance, how likely is it that this patient is adding interpretations into his own primary experience? If so, in what direction? How suggestible is the patient in the interview process? How consistent is the information reported when approached from different perspectives? How motivated is the patient to communicate a particular version of his narrative? Have direct questions been used to obtain certain information? With some ideas about the overlaid layers of information, is it possible to parse the current information to 'peel off' the overlaid layers, in order to gain a better sense of the information in the original experience in PM(t0)?

9.4 Handling Clinical Categories

In the clinical dialogue, *after* the major clarification of 'what' the patient is suffering from, the clinician has to decide upon how best to help the patient. At this stage, there is a point of transition from phenomenology to psychiatry.

In trying to decide about management, clinicians may follow 'heuristics' to decide on the best approach. A large number of objects and situations are grouped together into a smaller number of categories on the assumption that situations belonging to the same category require similar responses. There is thus a correspondence between the number of perceptual categories and the number of actionable responses. The number of categories is inherently related to the number of different possible responses. For instance, when there are many different possible responses, classification into a larger number of categories is necessary. Likewise, when the number of responses is limited, the number of perceptual categories will be smaller (Zwaan & Radvansky, 1998).

In mental health scenarios, this situation becomes challenging because the number of responses differs according to approaches taken by each practitioner. Different ways of conceiving and describing mental disorders have been attempted. They are not necessarily mutually exclusive. For instance, the categories that could be used to guide psychotherapeutic interventions may be different from those that are used to guide psychopharmacology interventions. Integrated consideration of both may be complementary and enriching.

Making a 'diagnosis' involves mapping the patient's condition into a category within a system of classification. One important level of categorization is the 'symptom classification' process. We note that symptom classification is used differently from phenomenological clarification. In the latter we characterize the individual details without assumptions. In symptom classification, we assume that the experience will map onto one of the known symptom prototypes, and the task is to make this mapping, for example, whether this patient has experienced a third-person auditory hallucination. This process is crucial to diagnosis; once symptom classification has been accomplished, diagnosis follows explicit, man-made rules according to the latest version of the classification system.

The symptom classification process involves comparing details of the anomalous psychopathology experience in the patient with those reported in other patients. As such, symptom classification reduces the complexity of the clinical information into membership of symptom categories. Categorization is widely used in human endeavours (Neisser, 1989). Often, membership in a category implies that similar outcomes are expected. A typical example involves diagnosis in internal medicine. Signs and symptoms are first identified. They lead to a diagnosis. Given a diagnosis, a management pathway follows (see Figure 9.3).

In medicine, a large amount of clinical information is funnelled into a categorical diagnostic formulation (Elstein & Schwarz, 2002). Given the same diagnostic categories, similar management pathways follow. Information at the level of symptoms is used only for arriving at the diagnosis and may not be further utilized in determining the management plan.

In psychopathology, comprehensive formulation often calls for more individualized considerations. Symptom clarification is only one source of information that leads to a multi-faceted management plan. Information about biographical details, social circumstances, personalities, and the Lifeworld inhabited by the patient is also important in informing the management plan. The 'funnelling' of information is less steep in mental health formulations compared with that in general medicine.

In decisions about clinical intervention for patients, we have to utilize the best possible existing empirical knowledge, however incomplete it is. In this situation, the clinician will construct a clinical *formulation* for the patient, linking the individual patient to existing knowledge about aetiology and treatment of the condition. The formulation can be suggested by three pragmatic clinical questions: (1) Why has this patient (and not others) developed anomalous experiences? (2) Why does he suffer from these particular mental experiences (rather than other ones)? (3) Why do these develop at

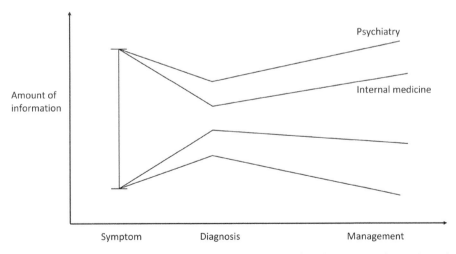

Figure 9.3. Schematic diagrams showing the informational roles of symptoms, diagnosis, and management in psychiatry and internal medicine. In both psychiatry and clinical medicine, diagnosis summarizes symptom information. In clinical medicine diagnosis plays a more critical role in that much of management would follow the diagnosis. In contrast, in psychiatry, although the diagnosis contains information relevant to clinical management, much of the clinical history is not subsumed under the diagnosis and is still directly relevant to the management plan (see section 9.4).

this time in the course of his or her life development (and not earlier)? The responses to these questions involve applying knowledge about the condition to the individual patient. We formulate hypotheses about why this clinical condition has arisen, given the constitutional and developmental features of that individual. Constructing a clinical formulation compels us to think about factors that may underlie the subject's condition and thereby identify key foci for intervention.

In this process too, the patient has to be understood as a person who is a developing agent, interacting actively with the environment (see section 4.1.1. on person development). It is also recognized that an individual does not exist in isolation but exists in relation to other individuals (see section 3.5.1 on relating). Adequate assessments therefore include both a longitudinal and a cross-sectional perspective, according to the model of the Person developed in the previous sections. In the longitudinal perspective, developmental changes over time are highlighted. Key processes involved in shaping the life course of the patient are identified. We note that these are similar to the domains we have covered in the phenomenological understanding of the patient, but this time the viewpoint is not from the patient's 'insider' perspective but from an 'outsider's' perspective, looking at objective environmental and developmental factors that are associated with the illness.

The clinician's application of clinical categories is an inherent process in a clinical interview, where action is expected as an outcome. However, premature application of these categories may mislead the psychopathological phenomenological evaluation. It is conceivable that under pressure of time constraints and cognitive constraints (e.g., with excessive caseloads), these important clinical processes may be compromised. Explicit articulation of the processes involved in psychopathological assessment may allow us to estimate the limits to which psychiatric assessments can be compressed without compromising their informational quality.

9.5 Unpacking Patient's Accounts

During a clinical interview, the patient develops an account of psychopathological experiences in the context of his life histories. The patient produces this account through verbal language. This process involves some re-organization of the primary subjective experiences.

Such accounts are sometimes referred to as 'narratives', to emphasize they are not always only concerned with depicting 'objective facts'. When the patient is narrating, he acknowledges his intentions and describes how he reacts to the perceived reality. For example, in a narrative medical account, the patient is often predominantly considered as an object of pathology and treatment but less often as an active agent responding to illness. As a result, there is a risk of under-recognizing the patient's choices and actions. The consequences of ignoring this domain are particularly undesirable in mental illness, where the patient's action often can play a crucial role.

9.5.1 Interpretations (verstehen)

9.5.1.1 Etic and emic descriptions

Psychopathology can be enriched by concepts from ethnography (a discipline developed to study human experiences in different populations and contexts). Ethnography has developed useful conceptual tools to facilitate empathic understanding of people's experiences in unfamiliar contexts. The two basic approaches of understanding have been designated as 'etic' and 'emic'. The etic approach investigates a social group from within, using shared concepts from within the group; the emic approach studies the group from the perspective of an outsider, using the framework of the outsider's meaning structure. In the study of psychopathology, it is assumed that the clinician shares socio-cultural background with the patients, and when this is not the case, special care needs to be taken to stay with the etic approach as much as possible.

9.5.1.2 Thick descriptions

In ethnography, 'thick description' has been employed in the study of human cultures (Geertz, 1973). It includes an account of not only a behaviour itself but importantly also its context. When context is included, the behaviour becomes culturally meaningful (see section 9.5 on context).

When investigators (whether an anthropologist or a clinician) try to understand their subjects' experiences, it is important that they should not uncritically assume that they can grasp the contextual information in the same way that their subject has experienced it. For the clinician it is desirable to first try to understand the subject's experience through concrete examples of shared meanings. In the process, the clinician will need to grasp the contexts in which the subject encounters his individual subjective experiences, not assuming that it will have perfect alignment with the clinician's own experiences. This process of understanding may involve identifying key terms used by the subject to describe experience and to grasp the meaning of such terms as used by the subject through exploring the Lifeworld contexts in which these terms have been used.

9.5.1.3 Accounts of psychopathological experiences as illness narratives

As a psychopathologist, the clinician takes into account the structural characteristics of illness stories and their relationships to individual life histories. Illness narratives are stories unfolding in time (Ricoeur, 1981), working towards resolutions. Receivers of illness stories receive them by re-composing the stories through their own representations (reader response theory, Iser, 1978). These processes are also embedded in the clinical dialogue and cannot be ignored. The psychopathologist needs to have an awareness of how the narrative structure has contributed to and infiltrated the account of the primary illness experience.

Is the primary experience accessible in a form immune from secondary elaborations (as in story telling)? Raw pre-narrated experiences are sometimes seen as fleeting, formless, ungraspable, and inaccessible. This is the realm of primary raw subjective experience that the psychopathologist attempts to access. However, our minds are also programmed to organize these raw experiences to generate some order through a narrative structure. Primary experiences are not immune from this process of making sense. To the person, meaning lies in the relationships amongst semantic elements involved in the narrative structure (Good, 1993). To the psychopathologist, the narrative overlaid upon the patient's account should be disentangled as far as possible from the account of the primary illness experience.

9.6 Techniques in the Clinical Dialogue

9.6.1 Ambience of the clinical dialogue

In this section, it will be demonstrated that, like any clinical examination, a thoughtful arrangement of essential items involved in the clinical dialogue process is important for the proper conduct of the psychopathological interview. Physical details often determine the psychological ambience.

The minimum set of items involved in the interview involves a small room in which at least two chairs are placed, one for the subject and one for the interviewer. It should be understood that how they are arranged can already have an impact on the interview process. Spatial arrangement of the two chairs involves alignment and distance. Two chairs placed too far apart will impede communication, as hearing becomes effortful. Two chairs placed too close together will impose an uncomfortable psychological proximity between the subject and the interviewer and can lead to a compensatory increase of psychological distance.

Alignment of the orientation between the two chairs in relation to one other is also a critical determinant of the psychological ambience for the clinical dialogue.

Two chairs that face one another in opposite directions will impose a direct face-to-face confrontation between the patient and the interviewer (see Figure 9.4). In this manner, the subject and the interviewer will have to make a deliberate effort in order not to look directly at one another. Participants in conversation often find this position uncomfortable. Studies have revealed that participants engaged in eye contact for only part of the time during a natural conversational process (Argyle, 1975). For example, eye contact is made more often during 'turn-taking' points in the dialogue process. It decreases after a turn-taking transition when participants are fully engaged in the contents of the verbal discourse. This naturalistic pattern of eye contact in the conversation can be disrupted by psychopathological processes. Therefore, the level of eye contact has conventionally been regarded as important in a clinical observation.

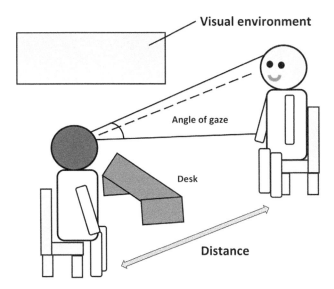

Figure 9.4. Space management in the clinical dialogue. The visual environment of the interview space, the distance between and alignments of the seats of the participants, and the presence and placement of a desk can influence the psychological ambience of the clinical dialogue (see section 9.6.1).

Seating positions in which the subject and the interviewer have to make deliberate efforts either to engage or to disengage eye contact compromise the sensitivity of this observation. It is therefore desirable in the naturalistic observational process that the chairs are aligned in a way that participants do not have to make exaggerated efforts, either to engage or to disengage from eye contact.

9.6.1.1 Chair arrangements: A

This arrangement reduces the eye contact (see Figure 9.5). The two persons look ahead of them with little eye contact. In this situation, the two persons have to make extra effort to make eye contact. This arrangement leads to increased psychological distance between the participants in an interview. While in general such distance makes the interview more impersonal, it may be a helpful feature for an extremely anxious patient talking about a sensitive topic.

9.6.1.2 Chair arrangements: B

The ideal alignment is between 90 and 180 degrees: The principle is that the participants should not need to make much extra effort either to look at or not to look at the other person (see Figure 9.6). The sensitivity for clinical observations on eye contact

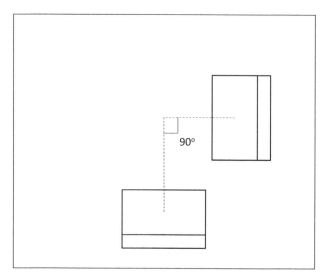

Figure 9.5. Chairs arrangements: A. In this arrangement, eye contact between the participants is minimized. This alignment is good when a more relaxed ambience is required to promote a more difficult conversation. It may compromise the clinician's observation of the subject (see section 9.6.1.1).

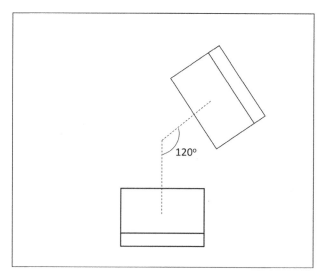

Figure 9.6. Chairs arrangements: B. In this arrangement, both participants can shift gaze easily, allowing the choice for maintaining eye contact or withdrawing from eye contact. This is the best position to observe the naturalistic amount of eye contact in the clinical dialogue (see section 9.6.1.2).

is higher if the persons have maximum freedom to choose whether or not to engage in eye contact.

9.6.1.3 *Positioning of the table*

The psychological effect of introducing a table in the room is that it represents a physical barrier. The barrier could signify an unequal relationship. Before we introduce the table, the space in the room is largely symmetrical. The table imposes an asymmetry that places the clinician and the patient into an unequal relationship (see Figure 9.7). Within this asymmetrical space, the clinician can view more of the patient while the patient can view less of the clinician. This creates an unequal 'observer versus observed' relationship. The table also suggests a protective barrier, creating a sense that one person is being protected more from the other. It is important to be aware that these spatial cues may influence the psychological ambience for the participants.

9.6.1.4 *Visual environment in the dialogue*

When a person enters a room, the room presents itself as the visual environment for the person. We normally do not pay much conscious attention to all the details of a visual environment. Instead we filter out irrelevant details and focus on the significant

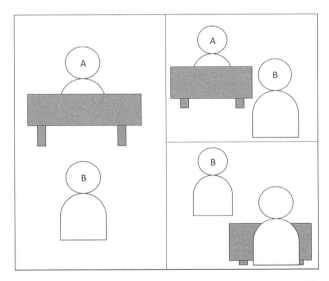

Figure 9.7. Positioning of the table. The psychological effect of placing a table pushes A and B into an unequal relationship. Left: A can observe more of B, compared with B's range of observation of A (lower right). This put A into the role of the observer more (see section 9.6.1.3).

details. In a patient with a mental disorder, often the capacity for attentional filtering is impaired. The patient may not be able to focus on key items but may instead become aware of a larger number of less relevant items in the room. In this paradoxical situation the patient may become more aware of certain aspects of the visual environment than the interviewer. This is because the interviewer has filtered out irrelevant features in the environment but the patient has not. This creates an interesting situation where the patient actually takes in some information from the immediate visual environment of the room that the clinician is not aware of. If the patient subsequently utilizes that information in the dialogue, the clinician may end up not being aware of this link. It would be advisable that a deliberate survey over the visual details in the room is made before the start of an interview.

9.6.1.5 *Accessories: Tissues and notes*

A box of tissues placed on the table is an effective symbol. In an interview, patients may be in touch with distressing emotions. Communication during these moments is often of high information value. However, at these moments, the patient often chooses to control his emotions out of embarrassment, by moving away from the topics that cause distress. In a supportive environment the patient should feel safe to experience the distress. If a box of tissues is available, the interviewer has the choice of offering the tissue in a graceful gesture of support.

Offering the patient a box of tissues signifies the clinician's readiness to go into emotional issues. Indeed, having the tissues ready from the beginning gives a visible signal that emotions are not to be shunned in the interview.

9.6.1.6 *Personal items (habitus)*

Personal accessories are visible items we carry with us, like jewellery or watches. Accessories are habitus that we have chosen, and therefore they contain information about ourselves. They are visible and informational to the patient. It is important to recognize that the clinical dialogue involves two interacting people. In this two-way process, the patient is also 'assessing' the clinician. Information from the clinician will to some extent determine the patient's behaviour. Through accessories, clinician's preference and values are perceived by the patient and influence the patient's communication with the clinician.

Personal items give information about the values, aesthetics, and choices of the clinician. This information can dichotomize patients into two groups: One group consists of patients who align with the clinician in their expressed values and the other group does not align with the clinician. If the patient perceives that the clinician does not share the same values, then the patient will have less confidence that the clinician can be empathic over his problems. Therefore, in general, clinicians should not unnecessarily draw attention to their personal values.

9.6.2 Directing the clinical dialogue

A repertoire of different interview styles is required to engage different patients. It is useful to consider two contrasting dialogue styles as reference poles. They are the checklist approach and the responsive approach (see Figure 9.8).

9.6.2.1 *Perception of control*

Control is a key concept in the clinical dialogue. 'Control' refers to the extent to which each participant determines the direction of the dialogue. The amount of clinician control within a particular interview needs to be managed carefully. Inadequate control from the clinician results in an ineffective interview. In an interview lacking in direction, the patient may not feel reassured with the professionalism of the interviewer. On the other hand, excessive control may result in the patient being passive, disengaged, or even defensive. A skilful clinician regulates control through the use of implicit transition gates between different topics in the interview (see section 9.7.2.3 on gate).

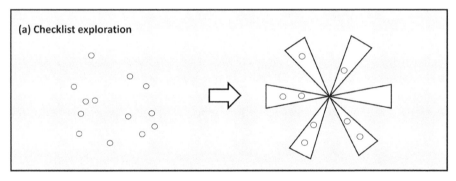

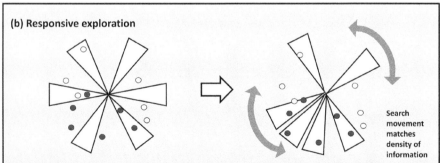

Figure 9.8. Explorations in checklist and responsive approaches. Top: checklist exploration; the regular spacing of observation sampling irrespective of emerging information enables a systematic, but less efficient exploration. Bottom: responsive exploration that allows more intense exploration in areas of higher complexity, resulting in a more efficient process (see section 9.6.2).

9.6.2.2 *The checklist approach*

The checklist approach covers a comprehensive list of questions in a predetermined order. Regardless of what the patient's response to the previous questions is, the next question follows in the same sequence. The checklist approach is used in a structured research interview. Coverage of the listed area is assured. However, the flexibility to explore specific areas in greater depth in response to unfolding information is limited.

9.6.2.3 *The responsive approach*

In the responsive approach, the questions raised by the clinicians are not predetermined. As in everyday dialogue, the next question is formulated based on the patient's previous response. The responsive approach results in a more natural flow of conversation. It allows for a more flexible exploration that can be adjusted in real time to be proportionate to the informational content of particular domains for the particular patient.

During the interview, the clinician regularly monitors rapport with the patient. The degree of rapport can be indicated by the alignment at verbal and non-verbal levels between the clinician and the patient. Indicators of rapport include the amount of verbal response, the engagement of shared attention in the dialogue, and various non-verbal indicators of dialogue alignment (see Figure 9.9 and section 9.6.3 on conversation alignment). A well-aligned dialogue proceeds in a smooth conversational flow with the relevant contents. The amount of elaboration is appropriately regulated, with participants giving just enough, but no more, information so that they can be understood (i.e., in compliance with the Grice's maxim). Non-verbal communication, as indicated by the

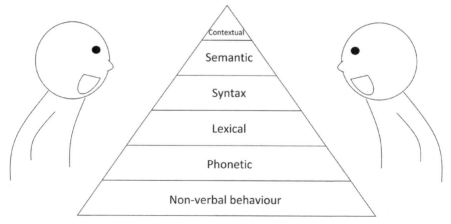

Figure 9.9. Levels of linguistic alignment in dialogue. From top to bottom: context, semantic, syntax, lexical, phonetic, and non-verbal levels. These levels are increasingly shared between participants in a dialogue as time goes by. More similarity is shared between the participants (see section 9.6.3).

level of eye contact as well as bodily gestures (e.g., inclination of the upper body when seated), also exhibits convergence between participants. Regular monitoring of these indicators enables the clinician to gauge whether rapport has increased or decreased during different stages of the interview.

9.6.3 Alignments in the clinical dialogue

In the clinical dialogue cycle (see section 9.3), interactive processes between the interviewer and the subject transfer information at different linguistic levels.

In the dialogue one person initiates the conversation by activating a context for the communication. Linguistic information expressed by the first participant sets up anticipatory activation of a cognitive structure in the second participant. This cognitive structure in the second participant is used to determine the response, which in turn activates a revision of the cognitive structure in the first participant. Thus, in iterations of conversations, the cognitive structures in the participants undergo a process of alignment. This interactive effect occurs at multiple linguistic levels. They include basic acoustic and phonemic levels as well as higher levels of syntax, semantics, and discourse.

At the phonetic level, the participants activate the cognitive structures that take into account the individual voice characteristics in order to decode the physical sound waves. This is a process of extracting information from a complex mixture of background and foreground sounds. Background information is relatively invariant (such as the background noises in the environment). Foreground information is phonemes that are rapidly changing and carry the informational contents. Embedded in the sound stream are also the relatively stable voice characteristics of the speaker.

Incoming physical sound waves are segregated automatically into streams. The assignment of sound characteristics into relatively invariant channels enables the decoding and more accurate extraction of information in the target phonemic channels (refer to difference-same comparison in section 6.3). In addition to the foreground informational content, the listener sets up a representation of the background information, which enables more efficient extraction of the foreground information in subsequent processes.

The process of setting up background (contextual) information constitutes part of the mechanisms for 'alignment' (Garrod & Pickering, 2009; Pickering & Garrod, 2004). Setting up representations for the invariant background information in a conversation results in an alignment of these representations for the participants as the conversation proceeds. Alignment occurs at different psycholinguistic levels. Apart from the phonetic level, similar processes occur at the syntactic, thematic, and discourse levels. At the syntactic level, aligned participants tend to use similar grammatical structures (referring to the order of the nouns, objects, and phrases within the sentence). The availability of this shared pattern is helpful for resolving syntactic ambiguity in the conversation (e.g., whether a particular word is being used as a verb or a noun). Similarly, at the semantic level, alignment occurs in word meanings. As many linguistic symbols have multiple interpretative possibilities, every instance of the use of a word involves some judgement as to the specific meaning that the word conveys in that particular context. During a dialogue cycle, contextual information is set up and shared between the participants. Alignment in the semantic context allows efficient communication between the participants with minimum redundancy. During the process of semantic alignment, participants are familiarized with the other person's choice of words and their associated meanings. A well-aligned conversation conveys complex information parsimoniously between the two participants. This phenomenon is summarized in the Grice's maxim (1975). In specific psychopathological conditions, dialogue alignment may be affected, leading to difficulty in grasping the context of the conversation.

In the alignment process, it should be noted that ideas can be conveyed from one individual to another without full explicit description (e.g., in the use of metaphors). In these situations, the recipient of the information is susceptible to influences based on his own inferred understanding. Misalignment as well as erroneous construal of representations can occur.

In everyday life, human communications occur with profound economy (e.g., Grice's maxim). However, this economy may cause specific difficulties in the assessment of psychopathology, as well as in the longitudinal 'acculturation' of the patients to medical terminology. Communication using a technical term without clear definition can have profound implications for patients. Similarly, clinicians may be tempted to uncritically accept a technical term used by the patient without clarifying the primary phenomenon. For instance, when a patient reports a particular experience as a 'dream', it would be prudent for a clinician to go into further details to clarify that the relevant phenomenon is indeed an experience that occurs in the dream state rather than, for instance, a hypnagogic state or, metaphorically, of a pleasant hope for the future.

Importantly, difficulty in alignment may actually provide information for the clinician as to the level of disorganization in the cognitive psycholinguistic structures in patients. As a result of mutual alignments, the clinician, immediately after talking to a patient with language disorganization, can experience subtle difficulty in organizing his own speech. If the clinician is aware of this change, he could use this observation to increase his sensitivity in detecting subtle language disorganization in the patient.

Under some circumstances, responses in the preceding part of the interview can have an impact on the immediately following part of the interview. The way in which a person responds to the same questions may vary according to the previous questions because of the different contexts that have been set up by the previous questions (see section 9.3). This leads to an important recognition that the 'line of approach' leading to the current questions may have a profound effect on the responses. Therefore, in the assessment of a psychopathological phenomenon, it is important that clinicians use different lines of approach in order to capture different perspectives from which a symptom can be explored. A reliance on a single 'line of approach' can result in information that is narrow and at times misleading. These realizations bring us back to an appreciation of the principle of uncertainty in which the act of the observation itself can have an impact on the phenomenon being observed.

9.7 Structure of the Clinical Dialogue

9.7.1 Parallel levels of interaction in the clinical dialogue

At any time during the interview, information flows at a number of different levels. There are three major levels. The first is the 'factual' level, in which an account is elaborated about the history and circumstances of the client. This information is historical-factual in nature and is considered in the context of a clinical dialogue with a narrative structure (see section 9.5 on narrative). At the same time there is the second level of 'psychopathology', in which the primary raw experience of potential symptoms is communicated by patients. When the interview focuses on this level, the clinician and patient engage in 'iterative clinical dialogue cycles' to clarify the symptoms (see section 9.3). At the same time that subjective experiences are clarified, observation of behaviour during the dialogue interaction also takes place (see section 1.2). The third level in the interview is the 'interpersonal' level. This refers to the interactional processes between the clinician and the patient. Engagement, empathic responses, dialogue alignments, negotiation of control, and so forth are processes that belong to this level. The clinician should be able to monitor key alignment variables in the interactional dimension as the interview proceeds. A particular dialogue can be located more at one level than another, and the response of the clinician can also focus the dialogue on a particular plane. For example, patients could be talking about an experience of auditory hallucinations on a particular evening. The clinician then has to decide whether to engage the dialogue at the historical-narrative level, in which case the follow-up question can be 'what happened before that?' or 'how did you respond to that experience?'. Alternatively, the clinician can choose to locate the dialogue at a symptom elaboration cycle, in which case the following question can be 'can you tell me more about those voices, what were they like exactly?'

9.7.2 Key stages in a clinical dialogue

It is useful to conceptualize distinct stages for an interview in order that different tasks can be the focus in different stages (see Figure 9.10, Shea, 1998). A thoughtful clinician carefully considers the timing for each task in the interview and weighs up the pros and cons for the different sequences in which the components can be completed. Skilful interviewers are also able to adjust and modify the sequence in real time according to needs. Awareness of the structure of the interview is important for strategic management of the interview (see section 9.7.2.1). Most interviews should contain at least three distinct sections: a beginning, a body, and an ending section.

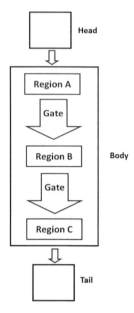

Figure 9.10. Stages of interview. From top to bottom: head, body (region A, B, and C), and tail. The head consists of initial explorations and observations. The body is where most of the content information takes place. The tail is for summing up and clarification (see section 9.7.2).

9.7.2.1 *Processes in the clinical dialogue*

9.7.2.1.1 Beginning

Initiating the clinical interview is a crucial process that is often not adequately managed. It is important for the clinician to set aside designated attention for the task in the first few minutes of the interview. Successful engagement in this stage enhances the effectiveness of the entire interview.

9.7.2.1.2 Sharing the context

A proper introduction to the context of the interview is of utmost importance. Introducing the situation (e.g., specifying the duration and purpose of the interview) clearly in the introductory phase enables the clinician and the patient to be engaged in a spirit of openness and equity. Equity in information exchange allows the patient to become an active participant in the process of the interview. This equity cannot be taken for granted because of the unequal power roles between the clinician and the patient in many cultures (Nimmon & Stenfors-Hayes, 2016). Implied in a competent

introduction process is the signal that the patient will be respected as an active participant in the clinical dialogue. A proper initiation avoids a coercive atmosphere in the
interview. In an asymmetrical relationship, a defensive attitude in the patient may arise
and impinge on the validity of the data obtained. The more the clinician shares control
with the subject, the better the clinician can engage the patient. If the patient is participating in a half-hearted manner, the validity of the emerging data will be compromised.
This is particularly important for anxious or defensive subjects. In these instances, it
is even more important to ensure that the subject experiences a sense of control over
the interview process. Sometimes, it is worth making an explicit statement to the effect
that 'Although this interview may touch on something distressing, I would like you to
know that you can stop the interview at any time. If you feel uncomfortable or there
are areas that you don't wish to talk about, please let me know and I will respect that.'
Giving this reassurance sometimes helps anxious patients to become more at ease and
less defensive.

9.7.2.1.3 Initial observation

One important task for the first few minutes in the interview is making initial observations about the appearance and behaviour of the patient. It is worthwhile setting aside
several minutes at the beginning of the interview to accomplish this observation. This
observation should be conducted at the beginning of the interview rather than at the
end for several reasons. At the beginning of the interview, the interviewer is still relatively sensitive to any unusual features in the patient's physical presentation. After the
interview has been in progress for some time, the clinician becomes heavily engaged in
the verbal content of the dialogue and can spare less attention on the visual details. In
addition, if an equivocal observation is made only at a later stage in the interview, there
is only limited time left for re-confirming the observation. In contrast, if the observation is made in the beginning of the interview, there are still opportunities for further
monitoring and further observation.

9.7.2.1.4 Screening for potential interview impasse

Another important task at the beginning of the interview is screening for potential
interview *impasse*. The first few minutes can be used as an exploration of the anticipated
pattern of the clinical dialogue. In this exploration, the clinician engages the patient in
a casual dialogue on a range of neutral, non-threatening topics. The clinician observes
the nature of this communication in order to generate some anticipation about how the
interview is likely to unfold subsequently. Tendencies towards difficult communication
patterns observed at this stage (such as a 'shut-down' interview, Roter & Hall, 2006;
Shea, 1998) will enable an adjustment of interview style at an early stage in the interview to address some of the anticipated difficulties.

9.7.2.1.5 Engagement

Engagement in the sense of building up a relationship in which both participants work towards an aligned goal (i.e., a therapeutic alliance) is another important objective for the initial stage of the interview. This involves aligning mutual understanding in arriving at common objectives both the patient and the clinician seek. This process, taken for granted in other medical consultations, often requires substantial skills and efforts in psychiatric scenarios. During this process, the clinician and the patient become aligned at various psycholinguistic levels (e.g., phonetic, syntactic, semantic levels) as dialogue participants. Successful engagement is a prerequisite for a successful interview.

9.7.2.1.6 Probing for hidden agenda

In the process of engagement and alignment, it is important for clinicians to recognize that patients' main concerns might be different from the clinicians' objectives. This is often referred to as the 'hidden agenda'. Some exploration and probing will be required for the clinicians to come to an understanding of what lies at the core of the patients' concerns and to try to align those objectives with the clinician's own objectives in order to ensure successful therapeutic alliance with the patient.

9.7.2.1.7 Identifying an effective feedback channel

One key objective for the first few minutes is to identify an effective feedback channel with the patient. In particular, this involves deciding on the relative role of the visual and verbal channels. The channel is for communicating feedback in the interview. It is important for the dialogue process that regular feedback from the clinician is provided while the patient is communicating his or her account. Deliberate attention to this process is important as some channels might be compromised. For instance, if the level of eye contact in the patient is limited, then the visual feedback channel could be compromised, and non-verbal gestures such as nodding may not provide effective feedback. In this circumstance, more deliberate use of verbal feedback may be required.

9.7.2.2 *Regions and gates*

The body of the interview can be conceptualized according to the key concepts of Regions and Gates (Shea, 1998). Regions refer to a coherent body of information whose parts are related to one another, such as 'mood states' or the 'family history'. Gates refer to points at the interview where there is a transition from one region to another. We can conceptualize the interview as consisting of a linear progression through a number of regions, with the transition from one region to another being conducted by gates (see Figure 9.11). It is important to note that the dialogue process within one region tends to be natural, and less explicit control is required to direct the conversation. However, in transition between one region and another, a clear change of

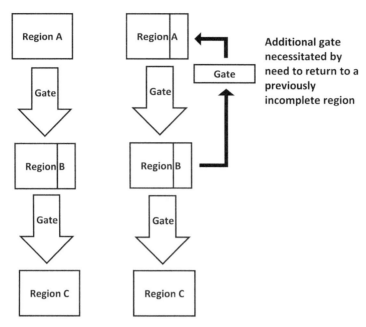

Figure 9.11. Regions and gates. A linear progression through regions (area of closely related information), with the transition from one region to another being conducted by gates. A gate is a transitional question leading to the conversation being moved to a different region. Within a region, dialogues can take place relatively freely. Transiting to a new region necessitates a change of direction. If the change is abrupt and direct, the atmosphere of the dialogue will move to being more like an interrogation, resulting in a less efficient process. Right: More gates are needed if regions are left prematurely, leaving a need to return subsequently (see section 9.7.2.3).

direction is often required. At this point, the issue of how control is negotiated between the clinician and the patient becomes a focus (see section 9.6.2.1 on control).

In a clinician-directed interview, the clinician imposes a gate transition in an explicit manner. For instance, the clinician might state 'We have finished talking about this area, let us change the topic to another area.' In this situation, the interview will acquire an ambience that is dominated by the clinician. The result is that the patient feels that his participation in the interview is less active. This may limit the free flow of information from the patient. A less directive interview style may encourage the patient to participate more in determining the content of the interview. In this case, the patient is allowed to take the lead to change towards different areas of discussion in the interview and the clinician will follow. This style will encourage the patient to be an active participant in the process and allows discussion in areas that the patient is concerned about. However, in some circumstances, for instance, when patients have disorganized communication, this style becomes less effective. In these scenarios the clinician will need to steer the dialogue more proactively.

An experienced clinician can provide direction without being explicitly domineering. Gate negotiation provides an excellent opportunity. If a clinician can pay attention to the process of transition from one region to another, he can often direct the transition in a way that feels less controlling. One notable way to achieve this is to link the first region with the second region using a bridging question. The bridging question provides a semantic link between the first and second regions. The clinician identifies the last area of exploration and then considers how these areas could be meaningfully linked to potential areas in the target region towards which he is seeking to move. After identifying the potential link, the clinician then formulates a question that provides a bridge in a natural manner. For example, the first area that has been explored is the 'mood state', and the second region that the clinician wishes to direct the interview may be to 'personality': The clinician can search the second region for a topic that is relatively close to the previous topic in the first region. For example, following an exploration of "mood state", an enquiry about drinking habits may become a possible point of entry. The clinician then tries to link the first region (mood state) with drinking, perhaps with a bridging question such as 'A lot of people will resort to drinking when they feel unhappy, I wonder what you think about this?' In this way, the patient will be guided to a conversation about drinking habits and then from the drinking habit an exploration of the rest of his lifestyle and personalities can be launched. Gate negotiation using a bridging question can be less explicitly directive and still focuses on a direction guided by the clinician.

Another general principle about regions and gates is that while the conversation stays in a region, the clinician should endeavour to explore the region fully before trying to move on to another region. Unnecessary moves between regions create the need for more gates as there is a need to return to the 'not-yet-fully-explored' first region at some points in the future. This unnecessarily increases the number of gates required in the interview session. The practice of fully exploring a region before moving on minimizes the number of gates in an interview session (see Figure 9.11).

9.7.2.3 *Empathic skills*

In fostering an empathic ambience for the interview, it is important to consider the provision of the right amount of psychological space. The issue with psychological space has already been discussed alongside physical spaces for the interview process (see section 9.6.1 on space). During the clinical dialogue, psychological space is important, particularly when considering the amount of empathic feedback the clinician gives to the subject. On the one hand, the interviewer may give very little feedback, thereby increasing the psychological distance. On the other hand, the interviewer can be offering too many feedback statements of empathy. This may result in intrusiveness and reduce the psychological space for patients. It is important to achieve the right balance between these positions.

9.7.2.3.1 Empathic statements

The explicit communication of empathy is important in the interview process. From time to time, the clinician gives signals to indicate that he has understood and empathizes with the patient's sharing. Such feedback can be simply acknowledging communication as discussed in the section on visual and verbal feedback (see section 9.7.2.1.7 on feedback channels). At other times, a more explicit statement of understanding, called 'empathic statement', is called for. An empathic statement is a verbal expression to the effect that the interviewer understands and appreciates what the patient has communicated. Empathic statements do not need to be made too often and should be made only after particularly significant sharing. An empathic statement can refer to factual content of what the patient had expressed, or it can reflect on the emotional implications of communication. Usually, empathic statements are qualified with varying degrees of certainty with phases such as 'it sounds like', 'it feels as if', or 'it must be'. It should be noted that for patients with psychotic symptoms, empathic statements can sometimes be interpreted as intrusive access to their mental state, and as such they can be perceived as threatening and may reinforce psychotic experiences (such as mind reading). The level of certainty to which an empathic statement is stated therefore needs to be qualified sensitively.

9.7.2.3.2 Here-and-now reflection

The 'here-and-now' reflection is a technique that brings the focus of the clinical dialogue to the present process of the interview itself. Often the content of an interview dialogue refers to events and experiences that have happened in the past outside the interview room. This external focus of the conversations is necessary to explore comprehensively what a person has experienced outside the interview setting. However, when the interview process itself becomes an important focus of attention, for example, when information flow is impeded in the interview, it may be necessary deliberately to focus on the 'here-and-now'. When it is necessary to bring the dialogue to the 'here-and-now', the psychological distance changes and the transition may be difficult for both the interviewer and the subject. In particular, the interviewer himself may feel threatened when the attention is turned to the interview process itself, as he needs to step forwards from a more hidden 'observer' position to come directly into view for possible discussion in the dialogue. The interviewer needs to overcome this reservation in order that the interview can freely proceed from the safer focus on 'there-and-then' to the more challenging focus on the 'here-and-now'. Notably, the 'here-and-now' reflection is used as a technique to address some interview difficulties (such as the shut-down interview, Shea, 1998).

9.8 Authenticity and Openness

The clinical dialogue is a unique encounter between two persons. To be effective, it requires the participants to be open to relate to the other person empathically. This purpose is best served with an open mind, with patience and attention to detail, minimizing assumptions. It allows the other person to go beyond one's expectations and to surprise. It also allows the other person to be creative in one's mind.

In this mode, the clinician is open to the possibility that the representational structure in his own mind can be changed by the encounter. The interview process becomes a creative interaction. Instead of being a closed one-way process, accommodation of new information is anticipated. This openness in authenticity will prevent a closure to new observations. This will address significant neglect over an area that could potentially yield useful information for advance in the understanding, recognition, and management of mental conditions.

A serious attempt to understand the distressing experiences of another person through empathy not only paves the way for better healing efforts but the encounter itself should make the suffering patient at least feel less isolated.

Conclusions

This work articulates a framework for contemporary psychopathology through an integration of biology, cognitive science, and phenomenology. It starts by examining the nature of psychopathological data as raw subjective experiences and ends with a pragmatic review of how to access quality phenomenological data in clinical settings. In this exploration, we are led to review our model of subjective experiences in the human person. This review highlights the need for a more comprehensive approach accommodating experiential as well as mechanistic perspectives. This approach addresses the shortcomings of a narrow mechanistic approach to mental illnesses.

This book asserts that subjective experiences (phenomena) of a person is of central importance to understanding mental illnesses. It also identifies the use of two key cognitive variables, information and representation, as crucial conceptual bridges between biology and phenomenology. Phenomenology and biology are complementary perspectives that can be integrated to construct a coherent account of human experiences and how it is affected by brain illnesses, as well as how the individual reacts to these experiences.

It is important to recognize that these perspectives should be integrated rather than polarized. Empathy is a key link between these elements. Empathy is also the basis upon which psychopathological evaluation becomes possible. The clinician needs to mobilize his own empathic processes to access psychopathology in another person. While this process allows some aspects of subjective experiences to be made shareable, it is important to be aware of its various limitations. Some of the limitations can be approached with a reflective process of clinical dialogue. Conceptual accounts of empathy can be integrated with empirical studies to yield a rich framework for understanding the processes involved in the practice of psychopathology.

This account lays the groundwork for innovative initiatives in the study of mental symptoms. It argues that some components of mental symptoms are shareable between individuals, consistent between individuals, and can be mapped to functions of the brain. The scientific foundation of such study gives the promise that the data will contain information at the level of brain-computational dysfunctions. Attention to these processes will enable the study of mental symptoms to discriminate better between different sources of anomalous processes that contribute to the evolution of symptoms. This will allow empirical data to be acquired in a more discerning manner. Such initiatives will require continuing efforts but will be rewarded with a more considered approach to the understanding of mental illnesses and a promise to contribute to better healing endeavours.

References

Introduction

Andrieu, B. (2006). Brains in the flesh: Prospects for a neurophenomenology. *Janus Head*, 9(3), 135–155.

Berrios, G. E. (1992). Phenomenology, psychopathology and Jaspers: A conceptual history. *History of Psychiatry*, 3(11), 303–327.

Berrios, G. E. (1994). The language of psychiatry: A time for a change? *Hong Kong Journal of Psychiatry*, 4, 5–10.

Berrios, G. E. (1996). *The history of mental symptoms: Descriptive psychopathology since the 19th century*. Cambridge University Press.

Fish, F. J., & Hamilton, M. (1985). *Fish's clinical psychopathology: Signs and symptoms in psychiatry* (2nd ed.). Wright.

Jaspers, K. (1963). *General psychopathology* (J. Hoenig & M. W. Hamilton, Trans.). Manchester University Press. (Original work published 1913)

Jaspers, K. (1968). The phenomenological approach in psychopathology. *British Journal of Psychiatry*, 114(516), 1313–1323. (Original work published 1912)

Marková, I. S., & Berrios, G. E. (1995). Mental symptoms: Are they similar phenomena? The problem of symptom heterogeneity. *Psychopathology*, 28(3), 147–157.

Marková, I. S., & Berrios, G. E. (2009). Epistemology of mental symptoms. *Psychopathology*, 28(3), 147–157.

Oyebode, F. (2015). *Sims' symptoms in the mind: Textbook of descriptive psychopathology* (5th ed.). Saunders Limited.

Stein, E. (1970). *On the problem of empathy* (W. Stein, Trans.). ICS Publications. (Original work published 1916)

Varela, F. J., & Shear, J. (1999). First-person methodologies: What, why, how. *Journal of Consciousness Studies*, 6(2–3), 1–14.

1. The Problem of Psychopathological Knowledge

Baars, B. J. (1997). *In the theater of consciousness: The workspace of the mind*. Oxford University Press.

Baars, B. J. (2002). The conscious access hypothesis: Origins and recent evidence. *Trends in Cognitive Sciences*, 6(1), 47–52.

Borsboom, D., Cramer, A. O., & Kalis, A. (2019). Brain disorders? Not really: Why network structures block reductionism in psychopathology research. *Behavioral and Brain Sciences, 42*, E2.

Crick, F. (1994). *The astonishing hypothesis: The scientific search for the soul.* Charles Scribner's Sons.

Critchley, S. (2001). *Continental philosophy: A very short introduction.* Oxford University Press.

Dilthey, W. (1961). *Gesammelte Schriften* (Vol. 5). Teubner Verlagsgesellschaft.

Fodor, J. A. (1968). *Psychological explanation: An introduction to the philosophy of psychology.* Random House.

Fodor, J. A. (1978). Propositional attitudes. *The Philosophy and Psychology of Cognition, 61*(4), 501–523.

Fodor, J. A. (1983). *The modularity of mind: An essay on faculty psychology.* MIT Press.

Geertz, C. (1973). *The interpretation of cultures: Selected essays.* Basic Books.

Husserl, E. (1954). *The crisis of the European sciences and transcendental phenomenology: An introduction to phenomenological philosophy* (D. Carr, Trans.). Northwestern University Press. (Original work published 1936)

Husserl, E. (1970). *Logical investigations* (2nd ed.) (J. N. Findlay, Trans.). Routledge. (Original work published 1913, 1921)

Jaspers, K. (1963). *General psychopathology* (J. Hoenig & M. W. Hamilton, Trans.). Manchester University Press. (Original work published 1913)

Kornhuber, H. H., & Deecke, L. (1965). Hirnpotentialänderungen bei Willkürbewegungen und passiven Bewegungen des Menschen: Bereitschaftspotential und reafferente Potentiale. *Pflüger's Archiv für die gesamte Physiologie des Menschen und der Tiere, 284*(1), 1–17.

Libet, B. (1985). Unconscious cerebral initiative and the role of conscious will in voluntary action. *Behavioral and Brain Sciences, 8*(4), 529–539.

Nowak, M. A., & Krakauer, D. C. (1999). The evolution of language. *Proceedings of the National Academy of Sciences, 96*(14), 8028–8033.

Popper, K. (1962). *Conjectures and refutations: The growth of scientific knowledge.* Basic Books.

Pylyshyn, Z. W. (1984). *Computation and cognition: Toward a foundation for cognitive science.* MIT Press.

Ryle, G. (1968). The thinking of thoughts: What is 'Le penseur' doing? In *Collected papers, II: Collected essays 1929–1968* (pp. 493–510). Hutchinson.

Schacter, D. L. (1989). On the relation between memory and consciousness: Dissociable interactions and conscious experience. In H. L. Roediger & F. I. M. Craik (Eds.), *Varieties of memory and consciousness: Essays in honour of Endel Tulving* (pp. 355–389). Erlbaum.

Searle, J. R. (1980). Minds, brains, and programs. *Behavioral and Brain Sciences, 3*(3), 417–424.

Searle, J. R. (1984). *Minds, brains and science.* Harvard University Press.

Solé, R. V., Corominas-Murtra, B., Valverde, S., & Steels, L. (2010). Language networks: Their structure, function, and evolution. *Complexity, 15*(6), 20–26.

Wang, L., Yu, C., Chen, H., Qin, W., He, Y., Fan, F., Zhang, Y., Wang, M., Li, K., Zang, Y., Woodward, T. S., & Zhu, C. (2010). Dynamic functional reorganization of the motor execution network after stroke. *Brain, 133*(4), 1224–1238.

Weber, M. (1968). *Economy and society* (G. Roth & C. Wittich, Trans.). University of California Press. (Original work published 1922)

2. Information in the Brain and Subjective Experiences

Abelson, R. P., Aronson, E. E., McGuire, W. J., Newcomb, T. M., Rosenberg, M. J., & Tannenbaum, P. H. (1968). *Theories of cognitive consistency: A sourcebook*. Rand McNally.

Adami, C., Ofria, C., & Collier, T. C. (2000). Evolution of biological complexity. *Proceedings of the National Academy of Sciences, 97*(9), 4463–4468.

Alós-Ferrer, C., & Farolfi, F. (2019). Trust games and beyond. *Frontiers in Neuroscience, 13*, 887.

Ananth, M. (2008). *In defense of an evolutionary concept of health: Nature, norms, and human biology*. Routledge.

Andrieu, B. (2006). Brains in the flesh: Prospects for a neurophenomenology. *Janus Head, 9*(3), 135–155.

Astington, J. W., & Jenkins, J. M. (1995). Theory of mind development and social understanding. *Cognition & Emotion, 9*(2–3), 151–165.

Baddeley, A. D., & Hitch, G. (1974). Working memory. In G. H. Bower (Ed.), *The psychology of learning and motivation: Advances in research and theory* (Vol. 8, pp. 47–89). Academic Press.

Baddeley, R., Hancock, P., & Földiák, P. (Eds.). (1999). *Information theory and the brain*. Cambridge University Press.

Barkow, J. H., Cosmides, L., & Tooby, J. (1992). *The adapted mind: Evolutionary psychology and the generation of culture*. Oxford University Press.

Bechtel, W., & Abrahamsen, A. (1991). *Connectionism and the mind: An introduction to parallel processing in networks*. Blackwell.

Bernard, C. (1974). *Lectures on the phenomena of life common to animals and plants* (H. E. Hoff, R. Guillemin, & L. Guillemin, Trans.). Charles C Thomas. (Original work published 1865)

Blackmore, S. (1999). *The meme machine*. Oxford University Press.

Bickerton, D. (1995). *Language and human behavior*. University of Washington Press.

Boyer, P. (2000). Evolution of the modern mind and the origins of culture: Religious concepts as a limiting-case. In P. Carruthers & A. Chamberlain (Eds.), *Evolution and the human mind: Modularity, language and meta-cognition* (pp. 93–112). Cambridge University Press.

Brooks, D. R., Wiley, E. O., & Brooks, D. R. (1988). *Evolution as entropy*. University of Chicago Press.

Buller, D. J. (2006). *Adapting minds: Evolutionary psychology and the persistent quest for human nature*. MIT Press.

Camerer, C. F. (2011). Dictator, ultimatum, and trust games. In *Behavioral game theory: Experiments in strategic interaction*. Princeton University Press.

Campbell, B. G. (1999). An outline of human phylogeny. In C. R. Peters & A. Lock (Eds.), *Handbook of human symbolic evolution* (pp. 31–52). Blackwell.

Colman, A. M. (2013). *Game theory and its applications: In the social and biological sciences*. Psychology Press.

Conkey, M. W. (1999). A history of the interpretation of European 'palaeolithic art': Magic, mythogram, and metaphors for modernity. In C. R. Peters & A. Lock (Eds.), *Handbook of human symbolic evolution* (pp. 288–349). Blackwell.

Crawford, C. (1998). Environments and adaptations: Then and now. In C. Crawford & D. L. Krebs (Eds.), *Handbook of evolutionary psychology: Ideas, issues, and applications* (pp. 275–302). Lawrence Erlbaum Associates.

Crawford, C., & Krebs, D. L. (Eds.). (1998). *Handbook of evolutionary psychology: Ideas, issues, and applications*. Lawrence Erlbaum Associates.

Cummins, D. D. (1996). Dominance hierarchies and the evolution of human reasoning. *Minds and Machines, 6*(4), 463–480.

Davies, P. (1999). *The fifth miracle*. Simon and Schuster.

Dawkins, R. (1976). *The selfish gene*. Oxford University Press.

Dawkins, R. (1982). *The extended phenotype*. Oxford University Press.

Dessalles, J. (2000). Language and hominid politics. In C. Knight, M. Studdert-Kennedy, & J. R. Hurford (Eds.), *The evolutionary emergence of language: Social function and the origins of linguistic form* (pp. 62–80). Cambridge University Press.

Dietrich, E. (2007). Representation. In P. Thagard (Ed.), *Philosophy of psychology and cognitive science* (pp. 1–29). North-Holland.

Dretske, F. (1981). *Knowledge & the flow of information*. MIT Press.

Dunbar, R. (1996). *Grooming, gossip and the evolution of language*. Harvard University Press.

Dunbar, R. (1998). Theory of mind and the evolution of language. In J. R. Hurford, M. Studdert-Kennedy, & C. Knight (Eds.), *Approaches to the evolution of language: Social and cognitive bases* (pp. 148–166). Cambridge University Press.

Festinger, L. (1962). *A theory of cognitive dissonance* (Vol. 2). Stanford University Press.

Feynman, R. P., Leighton, R. B., & Sands, M. (1963). *The Feynman lectures on physics, Vol. I: The new millennium edition: Mainly mechanics, radiation, and heat* (Vol. 1). Basic Books.

Fodor, J. A. (1983). *The modularity of mind: An essay on faculty psychology*. MIT Press.

Franks, B., & Rigby, K. (2005). Deception and mate selection: Some implications for relevance and the evolution of language. In M. Tallerman (Ed.), *Language origins: Perspectives on evolution* (pp. 208–229). Oxford University Press.

Gleick, J. (2011). *The information: A history, a theory, a flood*. Pantheon Books.

Goldstein, K. (1939). *The organism: A holistic approach to biology derived from pathological data in man*. American Book Publishing.

Goodall, J. (1986). *The chimpanzees of Gombe: Patterns of behavior*. Bellknap Press of the Harvard University Press.

Harari, Y. N. (2014). *Sapiens: A brief history of humankind*. Harper. (Original work published 2011)

Hebb, D. O. (1949). *The organization of behavior*. Wiley.

Higginson, A. D., McNamara, J. M., & Houston, A. I. (2016). Fatness and fitness: Exposing the logic of evolutionary explanations for obesity. *Proceedings of the Royal Society, 283*(1822).

Holloway, R. (1999). Evolution of the human brain. In C. R. Peters & A. Lock (Eds.), *Handbook of human symbolic evolution* (pp. 74–125). Blackwell.

Hurford, J. R. (2003). The neural basis of predicate-argument structure. *Behavioral and Brain Sciences, 26*(3), 261–283.

Janis, I. (1982). *Groupthink: Psychological studies of policy decisions and fiascoes*. Houghton Mifflin.

Jaspers, K. (1963). *General psychopathology* (J. Hoenig & M. W. Hamilton, Trans.). Manchester University Press. (Original work published 1913)

Jensen, J., Smith, A. J., Willeit, M., Crawley, A., Mikulis, D. J., Vitcu, I., & Kapur, S. (2006). Separate brain regions code for salience vs. valence during reward prediction in humans. *Human brain mapping, 28*(4), 294–302.

Johnson-Laird, P. N. (1983). *Mental models: Towards a cognitive science of language, inference, and consciousness*. Harvard University Press.

Joordens, J. C., d'Errico, F., Wesselingh, F. P., Munro, S., De Vos, J., Wallinga, J., Ankjærgaard, C., Reimann, T., Wijbrans, J. R., Kuiper, K. F., Mücher, H. J., Coqueugniot, H., Prié, V., Joosten, I., Van Os, B., Schulp, A. S., Panuel, M., van der Haas, V., Lustenhouwer, W., . . . Roebroeks, W. (2015). Homo erectus at Trinil on Java used shells for tool production and engraving. *Nature, 518*(7538), 228–231.

Kahneman, D. (2011). *Thinking, fast and slow*. Macmillan.

Kempson, R. M. (Ed.). (1988). *Mental representations: The interface between language and reality*. CUP Archive.

Knight, C. (1998). Ritual/speech coevolution: A solution to the problem of deception. In J. R. Hurford, M. Studdert-Kennedy, & C. Knight (Eds.), *Approaches to the evolution of language: Social and cognitive bases* (pp. 68–91). Cambridge University Press.

Kosslyn, S. M. (1980). *Image and mind*. Harvard University Press.

Krause, L., Enticott, P. G., Zangen, A., & Fitzgerald, P. B. (2012). The role of medial prefrontal cortex in theory of mind: A deep rTMS study. *Behavioural Brain Research, 228*(1), 87–90.

Krebs, D. L. (1998). The evolution of moral behaviors. In C. Crawford & D. L. Krebs (Eds.). *Handbook of evolutionary psychology: Ideas, issues, and applications* (pp. 337–368). Lawrence Erlbaum Associates.

Kuhn, T. S. (1962). *The structure of scientific revolutions*. University of Chicago Press.

Lock, A., & Symes, K. (1999). Social relations, communication, and cognition. In C. R. Peters & A. Lock (Eds.), *Handbook of human symbolic evolution* (pp. 204–235). Blackwell.

Markman, A. B., & Dietrich, E. (2000). In defense of representation. *Cognitive Psychology, 40*(2), 138–171.

Marr, D. (1982). *Vision: A computational investigation into the human representation and processing of visual information*. MIT Press.

Maslow, A. H. (1943). A theory of human motivation. *Psychological Review, 50*(4), 370–396.

Miller, G. (1956). The magical number seven, plus or minus two: Some limits on our capacity for processing information. *The Psychological Review, 63*, 81–97.

Minsky, M. (1974). A framework for representing knowledge. In P. H. Winston (Ed.), *The psychology of computer vision*. McGraw-Hill.

Morris, R. G. M. (1989). Computational neuroscience: Modelling the brain. In *Parallel distributed processing: Implications for psychology and neurobiology* (pp. 203–213). Clarendon Press.

Moscovitch, M. (1995). Confabulation. In D. L. Schacter, J. T. Coyle, G. D. Fischbach, M. M. Mesulum, & L. G. Sullivan (Eds.), *Memory distortion* (pp. 226–251). Harvard University Press.

Newell, A., & Simon, H. (1976). Computer science as empirical inquiry: Symbols and search. *Communications of the ACM, 19*, 113–126.

Noble, J. (2000). Cooperation, competition and the evolution of prelinguistic communication. In C. Knight, M. Studdert-Kennedy, & J. R. Hurford (Eds.), *The evolutionary emergence of language: Social function and the origins of linguistic form* (pp. 40–61). Cambridge University Press.

O'Brien, E. J., Rizzella, M. L., Albrecht, J. E., & Halleran, J. G. (1998). Updating a situation model: A memory-based text processing view. *Journal of Experimental Psychology: Learning, Memory, and Cognition, 24*(5), 1200.

Pine, B. J., & Gilmore, J. H. (2011). *The experience economy*. Harvard Business Press.

Pinker, S. (2010). *The language instinct: How the mind creates language* (M. Hofmeisterova, Trans.). Penguin Books. (Original work published 1994)

Plotkin, J. B., & Nowak, M. A. (2000). Language evolution and information theory. *Journal of Theoretical Biology, 205*(1), 147–159.

Prigogine, I. (1967). *Introduction to thermodynamics of irreversible processes* (3rd ed.). Interscience.

Pylyshyn, Z. W. (1984). *Computation and cognition: Toward a foundation for cognitive science.* MIT Press.

Roese, N. J. (1994). The functional basis of counterfactual thinking. *Journal of Personality and Social Psychology, 66*(5), 805.

Rothbart, M. K., & Posner, M. I. (2007). *Educating the human brain.* American Psychological Association.

Rumelhart, D. E., McClelland, J. L., & PDP Research Group. (1987). *Parallel distributed processing.* MIT Press.

Shannon, C. E. (1948). A mathematical theory of communication. *The Bell System Technical Journal, 27,* 379–423.

Shapley, R. (1995). Parallel neural pathways and visual function. In M. S. Gazzaniga (Ed.), *The cognitive neurosciences* (pp. 315–324). MIT Press.

Smolensky, P. (1988). On the proper treatment of connectionism. *Behavioral and brain sciences, 11*(1), 1–23.

Smolensky, P. (1995). Reply: Constituent structure and explanation in an integrated connectionist/symbolic cognitive architecture. In C. MacDonald & G. MacDonald (Eds.), *Connectionism: Debates on psychological explanation* (Vol. 2, pp. 223–290). Blackwell.

Stark, L., & Theodoridis, G. C. (1973). Information theory in physiology. *Engineering principles in physiology, 1,* 13–32.

Swenson, R., & Turvey, M. T. (1991). Thermodynamic reasons for perception–action cycles. *Ecological Psychology, 3*(4), 317–348.

Talmi, D., Atkinson, R., & El-Deredy, W. (2013). The feedback-related negativity signals salience prediction errors, not reward prediction errors. *Journal of Neuroscience, 33*(19), 8264–8269.

Thompson, V. A., & Byrne, R. M. (2002). Reasoning counterfactually: Making inferences about things that didn't happen. *Journal of Experimental Psychology: Learning, Memory, and Cognition, 28*(6), 1154.

Tomasello, M., & Call, J. (1997). *Primate cognition.* Oxford University Press.

Tomasello, M., Carpenter, M., Call, J., Behne, T., & Moll, H. (2005). Understanding and sharing intentions: The origins of cultural cognition. *Behavioral and Brain Sciences, 28*(5), 675–735.

Ts'o, D. Y., & Roe, A. W. (1995). Functional compartments in visual cortex: Segregation and interaction. In M. S. Gazzaniga (Ed.), *The cognitive neurosciences* (pp. 325–337). MIT Press.

Turing, A. (1950). Computing machinery and intelligence. *Mind, 59*(236), 433–460.

Umeda, S., Mimura, M., & Kato, M. (2010). Acquired personality traits of autism following damage to the medial prefrontal cortex. *Social Neuroscience, 5*(1), 19–29.

Uomini, N. T., & Meyer, G. F. (2013). Shared brain lateralization patterns in language and Acheulean stone tool production: A functional transcranial Doppler ultrasound study. *PLoS One, 8*(8).

Wernicke, C. (2005). *An outline of psychiatry in clinical lectures: The lectures of Carl Wernicke* (R. Miller, & J. Dennison, Eds.). Springer. (Original work published 1881)

Wilson, E. O. (2012). *The social conquest of earth.* London: Liveright.

Worden, R. (1998). The evolution of language from social intelligence. In J. R. Hurford, M. Studdert-Kennedy, & C. Knight (Eds.), *Approaches to the evolution of language: Social and cognitive bases* (pp. 148–166). Cambridge University Press.

World Health Organization. (1948). *Frequently asked questions*. Retrieved from http://www.who.int/suggestions/faq/en/

Wynn, T. G. (1999). The evolution of tools and symbolic behaviour. In C. R. Peters & A. Lock (Eds.), *Handbook of human symbolic evolution* (pp. 261–287). Blackwell.

Yu, C. T. (1988). *Being and relation: A theological critique of western dualism and individualism (theology and science at the frontiers of knowledge)*. Scottish Academic Press.

Zwaan, R. A., & Radvansky, G. A. (1998). Situation models in language comprehension and memory. *Psychological Bulletin, 123*(2), 162.

3. The Structure of Subjective Experience

Brentano, F. (1973). *Psychology from an empirical standpoint* (L. L. McAlister, A. C. Rancurello, & D. B. Terrell, Trans.). Routledge. (Original work published 1874)

Buber, M. (1937). *I and thou* (R. G. Smith, Trans.). T&T Clark. (Original work published 1925)

Card, O. S. (1998). *Elements of fiction writing: Characters and viewpoint*. Writer's Digest Books.

Descartes, R. (1983). *Principles of philosophy* (V. Rodger & R. P. Miller, Trans.). D. Reidel. (Original work published 1644)

Dietrich, E. (2007). Representation. In P. Thagard (Ed.), *Philosophy of psychology and cognitive science* (pp. 1–29). North-Holland.

Eco, U. (1983). *The name of the rose* (W. Weaver, Trans.). Harcourt. (Original work published 1980)

Hnat Hanh, T. (1967). *Being peace*. Parallax Press.

Hnat Hanh, T. (1991). *The miracle of mindfulness*. Rider Books.

Husserl, E. (1970). *Logical investigations* (2nd ed.) (J. N. Findlay, Trans.). Routledge. (Original work published 1913, 1921)

James, W. (1890). *The principles of psychology*. Henry Holt.

Kabat-Zinn, J. (1990). *Full catastrophe living: Using the wisdom of your body and mind to face stress, pain, and illness*. Delta.

Pfander, A. (1900). *Phänomenologie des Wollens: Eine psychologische Analyse*. J.A. Barth.

Reinach, A. (1969). Concerning Phenomenology. (D. Willard, Trans.). *The Personalist, 50*, 194–211. (Original work published 1921).

Ritzel, H. (1916). Über analytische Urteile. Eine Studie zur Phänomenologie des Begriffs. *Jahrbuch für Philosophie Und Phänomenologische Forschung, 3*, 253–344.

Rosch, E. H. (1973). Natural categories. *Cognitive Psychology, 4*(3), 328–350.

Rosch, E. H. (1975). Cognitive representations of semantic categories. *Journal of Experimental Psychology: General, 104*(3), 192–233.

Sahn, S. (1976). *Dropping ashes on the Buddha* (S. Mitchell, Trans.). Grove Press.

Skinner, B. F. (1938). *The behavior of organisms: An experimental analysis*. Appleton-Century-Crofts.

St. Augustine of Hippo. (2012). *On the trinity* (P. A. Boer, Ed. & W. G. T. Shedd, Trans.). CreateSpace Independent Publishing Platform. (Original work published AD 400)

Stein, E. (1970). *On the problem of empathy* (W. Stein, Trans.). ICS Publications. (Original work published 1916)

Stein, E. (1998). *Potency and act: Studies toward a philosophy of being* (W. Redmond, Trans.). ICS Publications. (Original work published 1931)

Tomasello, M., & Call, J. (1997). *Primate cognition.* Oxford University Press.

Tomasello, M., Carpenter, M., Call, J., Behne, T., & Moll, H. (2005). Understanding and sharing intentions: The origins of cultural cognition. *Behavioral and Brain Sciences, 28*(5), 675–735.

4. Unfolding Phenomenological Processes in the Human Person

Amit, D. (1989). *Modeling brain function: The world of attractor neural networks.* Cambridge University Press.

Andreoli, V. (1996). *Carlo a mad painter. X World Congress of Psychiatry* (B. Jones, Trans.). Marsilio.

Andrieu, B. (2006). Brains in the flesh: Prospects for a neurophenomenology. *Janus Head, 9*(3), 135–155.

Brandom, R. (1979). Freedom and constraint by norms. *American Philosophical Quarterly, 16*(3), 187–196.

Buber, M. (1937). *I and thou* (R. G. Smith, Trans.). T&T Clark. (Original work published 1925)

Card, O. S. (1998). *Elements of fiction writing: Characters and viewpoint.* Writer's Digest Books.

Conkey, M. W. (1999). A history of the interpretation of European 'palaeolithic art': Magic, mythogram, and metaphors for modernity. In C. R. Peters & A. Lock (Eds.), *Handbook of human symbolic evolution* (pp. 288–349). Blackwell.

Földiák, P. (2002). Sparse coding in the primate cortex. In M. A. Arbib (Ed.), *The handbook of brain theory and neural networks* (2nd ed., pp. 1064–1068). MIT Press.

Hegel, G. W. F. (1977). *The phenomenology of spirit* (A. V. Miller, Trans.). Clarendon Press. (Original work published 1807)

Klyubin, A. S., Polani, D., & Nehaniv, C. L. (2008). Keep your options open: An information-based driving principle for sensorimotor systems. *PloS one, 3*(12).

Jaspers, K. (1963). *General psychopathology* (J. Hoenig & M. W. Hamilton, Trans.). Manchester University Press. (Original work published 1913)

Macquarrie, J. (1972). *Existentialism.* Westminster.

Piaget, J., & Inhelder, B. (1969). *The psychology of the child* (H. Weaver, Trans.). Basic Books.

Pine, B. J., & Gilmore, J. H. (2011). *The experience economy.* Harvard Business Press.

Stein, E. (1970). *On the problem of empathy* (W. Stein, Trans.). ICS Publications. (Original work published 1916)

Stein, E. (1998). *Potency and act: Studies toward a philosophy of being* (W. Redmond, Trans.). ICS Publications. (Original work published 1931)

Wernicke, C. (2005). *An outline of psychiatry in clinical lectures: The lectures of Carl Wernicke* (R. Miller, & J. Dennison, Eds.). Springer. (Original work published 1881)

Wynn, T. G. (1999). The evolution of tools and symbolic behaviour. In C. R. Peters & A. Lock (Eds.), *Handbook of human symbolic evolution* (pp. 261–287). Blackwell.

5. Empathic Access to Other People

Bayer, H. M., & Glimcher, P. W. (2005). Midbrain dopamine neurons encode a quantitative reward prediction error signal. *Neuron, 47*(1), 129–141.

Colman, A. M. (2013). *Game theory and its applications: In the social and biological sciences.* Psychology Press.

Corlett, P. R., Murray, G. K., Honey, G. D., Aitken, M. R., Shanks, D. R., Robbins, T. W., Bullmore, E. T., Dickinson, A., & Fletcher, P. C. (2007). Disrupted prediction-error signal in psychosis: Evidence for an associative account of delusions. *Brain, 130*(9), 2387–2400.

di Pellegrino, G., Fadiga, L., Fogassi, L., Gallese, V., & Rizzolatti, G. (1992). Understanding motor events: A neurophysiological study. *Experimental Brain Research, 91*, 176–180.

Eco, U. (1983). *The name of the rose* (W. Weaver, Trans.). Harcourt. (Original work published 1980)

Holroyd, C. B., & Coles, M. G. (2002). The neural basis of human error processing: Reinforcement learning, dopamine, and the error-related negativity. *Psychological Review, 109*(4), 679–709.

Husserl, E. (1970). *Logical investigations* (2nd ed.) (J. N. Findlay, Trans.). Routledge. (Original work published 1913, 1921)

Jaspers, K. (1963). *General psychopathology* (J. Hoenig & M. W. Hamilton, Trans.). Manchester University Press. (Original work published 1913)

Kant, I. (1998). *Critique of pure reason* (P. Guyer, & A. Wood, Eds.). Cambridge University Press. (Original work published 1781)

Lipps, T. (1903). Empathy, inner imitation and sense-feelings. In M. Rader (Ed.), *A modern book of esthetics* (pp. 374–382). Holt, Rinehart and Winston.

McDougall, W. (1908). The principal instincts and the primary emotions of man. In *An introduction to social psychology* (pp. 45–89). Methuen.

Meltzoff, A. N. (1994). Apprehending the intentions of others: Re-enactment of intended acts by 18-month-old children. *Developmental Psychology, 31*(5), 838–850.

Piaget, J., & Inhelder, B. (1969). *The psychology of the child* (H. Weaver, Trans.). Basic Books.

Preston, S. D., & De Waal, F. B. M. (2002). Empathy: Its ultimate and proximate bases. *Behavioral and Brain Sciences, 25*(1), 1–20.

Schultz, W. (2007). Behavioral dopamine signals. *Trends in Neurosciences, 30*(5), 203–210.

Solé, R. V., Corominas-Murtra, B., Valverde, S., & Steels, L. (2010). Language networks: Their structure, function, and evolution. *Complexity, 15*(6), 20–26.

Stein, E. (1970). *On the problem of empathy* (W. Stein, Trans.). ICS Publications. (Original work published 1916)

Titchener, E. B. (1909). *Lectures of the experimental psychology of thought processes.* Macmillan.

Zacks, J. M. (2008). Neuroimaging studies of mental rotation: A meta-analysis and review. *Journal of Cognitive Neuroscience, 20*(1), 1–19.

6. Mental Representations as Containers for Information in Subjective Experiences

Amit, D. (1989). *Modeling brain function: The world of attractor neural networks.* Cambridge University Press.

Andrieu, B. (2006). Brains in the flesh: Prospects for a neurophenomenology. *Janus Head, 9*(3), 135–155.

Aristotle. (1999). *Aristotle's metaphysics* (J. Sachs, Trans.). Green Lion Press.

Astington, J. W., & Jenkins, J. M. (1995). Theory of mind development and social understanding. *Cognition & Emotion*, 9(2–3), 151–165.

Barth, K. (1961). *Church dogmatics*. Westminster. (Original work published 1957)

Bliss, T. V., & Lomo, T. (1973). Long-lasting potentiation of synaptic transmission in the dentate area of the anaesthetized rabbit following stimulation of the perforant path. *Journal of Physiology*, 232(2), 331–356.

Borges, J. L. (1962). The library of Babel. In D. A. Yates & J. E. Irby (Eds.), *Labyrinths: Selected stories and other writings* (pp. 58–64). New Directions Publishing. (Original work published 1941)

Bregman, A. S. (1990). *Auditory scene analysis*. MIT Press.

Buber, M. (1937). *I and thou* (R. G. Smith, Trans.). T&T Clark. (Original work published 1925)

Bubic, A., Von Cramon, D. Y., & Schubotz, R. I. (2010). Prediction, cognition and the brain. *Frontiers in Human Neuroscience*, 4, 25.

Buckner, R. L., Andrews-Hanne, J. R., & Schacter, D. L. (2008). The brain's default network: Anatomy, function, and relevance to disease. *Annals of the New York Academy of Sciences*, 1124, 1–38.

Callard, F., & Margulies, D. S. (2014). What we talk about when we talk about the default mode network. *Frontiers in Human Neuroscience*, 8, 619.

Carruthers, G. (2007). A model of the synchronic self. *Consciousness and Cognition*, 16, 533–550.

Chechik, G., Meilijson, I., & Ruppin, E. (1998). Synaptic pruning in development: A computational account. *Neural Computation*, 10(7), 1759–1777.

Chen, E. Y. H. (1994). A neural network model of cortical information processing in schizophrenia. I: Interaction between biological and social factors in symptom formation. *The Canadian Journal of Psychiatry*, 39(8), 362–367.

Chen, E. Y. H. (1995). A neural network model of cortical information processing in schizophrenia. II: Role of hippocampal-cortical interaction: A review and a model. *The Canadian Journal of Psychiatry*, 40(1), 21–26.

Cheour, M., Ceponiene, R., Lehtokoski, A., Luuk, A., Allik, J., Alho, K., & Näätänen, R. (1998). Development of language-specific phoneme representations in the infant brain. *Nature Neuroscience*, 1(5), 351–353.

Colman, A. M. (2013). *Game theory and its applications: In the social and biological sciences*. Psychology Press.

Craik, F. I., & Bialystok, E. (2006). Cognition through the lifespan: Mechanisms of change. *Trends in Cognitive Sciences*, 10(3), 131–138.

Crews, F., He, J., & Hodge, C. (2007). Adolescent cortical development: A critical period of vulnerability for addiction. *Pharmacology Biochemistry and Behavior*, 86(2), 189–199.

Damasio, A. R. (1994). *Descartes' error: Emotion, reason and the human brain*. Putnam.

Damasio, A. R. (1996). The somatic marker hypothesis and the possible functions of the prefrontal cortex. *Philosophical Transactions: Biological Sciences*, 351(1346), 1413–1420.

David, N., Newen, A., & Vogeley, K. (2008). The 'sense of agency' and its underlying cognitive and neural mechanisms. *Consciousness and Cognition*, 17(2), 523–534.

de Bono, E. (1970). *Lateral thinking: Creativity step by step*. Harper Colophon.

Deacon, T. W. (1997). *The symbolic species: The co-evolution of language and the brain*. W. W. Norton & Company.

DeWitt, I., & Rauschecker, J. P. (2012). Phoneme and word recognition in the auditory ventral stream. *Proceedings of the National Academy of Sciences, 109*(8), E505–E514.

Dunbar, R. (1996). *Grooming, gossip and the evolution of language.* Harvard University Press.

Eilan, N., Marcel, A., & Bermúdez, J. L. (1995). Self-consciousness and the body: An interdisciplinary introduction. In J. L. Bermúdez, A. J. Marcel, & N. Eilan (Eds.), *The body and the self* (pp. 1–28). MIT press.

Eubank, L., & Gregg, K. (1999). Critical periods and (second) language acquisition: Divide et impera. In D. Birdsong (Ed.), *Second language acquisition and the critical period hypothesis* (pp. 65–99). Lawrence Erlbaum Associates.

Fauconnier, G., & Turner, M. (2008). *The way we think: Conceptual blending and the mind's hidden complexities.* Basic Books.

Forabosco, G. (1992). Cognitive aspects of the humor process: The concept of incongruity. *Humor-International Journal of Humor Research, 5*(1–2), 45–68.

Fung, Y. L. (1958). *A short history of Chinese philosophy* (D. Bodde, Trans.). Macmillan.

Fuster, J. M. (1990). Prefrontal cortex and the bridging of temporal gaps in the perception-action cycle. *Annals of the New York Academy of Sciences, 608*(1), 318–336.

Fuster, J. M. (2002). Physiology of executive functions: The perception-action cycle. In D. T. Stuss & R. T. Knight (Eds.), *Principles of frontal lobe function* (pp. 96–108). Oxford University Press.

Fuster, J. M. (2004). Upper processing stages of the perception–action cycle. *Trends in Cognitive Sciences, 8*(4), 143–145.

Gallagher, S. (2000). Philosophical conceptions of the self: Implications for cognitive science. *Trends in Cognitive Sciences, 4*(1), 14–21.

Gallese, V., & Goldman, A. (1998). Mirror neurons and the simulation theory of mind reading. *Trends in Cognitive Sciences, 12*, 493–501.

Gallese, V., Keysers, C., & Rizzolatti, G. (2004). A unifying view of the basis of social cognition. *Trends in Cognitive Sciences, 8*, 396–403.

Gallup, G. G., Platek, S. M., & Spaulding, K. N. (2014). The nature of visual self-recognition revisited. *Trends in Cognitive Sciences, 18*(2), 57–58.

Geertz, C. (1973). Religion as a cultural system. In *The interpretation of cultures: Selected essays* (pp. 87–125). Basic Books.

Goldstein, K. (1939). *The organism: A holistic approach to biology derived from pathological data in man.* American Book Publishing.

Haggard, P., Clark, S., & Kalogeras, J. (2002). Voluntary action and conscious awareness. *Nature Neuroscience, 5*(4), 382.

Hartshorne, J. K., Tenenbaum, J. B., & Pinker, S. (2018). A critical period for second language acquisition: Evidence from 2/3 million English speakers. *Cognition, 177*, 263–277.

Haslam, N. (2006). Dehumanization: An integrative review. *Personality and Social Psychology Review, 10*(3), 252–264.

Hegel, G. W. F. (1977). *The phenomenology of spirit* (A. V. MIller, Trans.). Clarendon Press. (Original work published 1807)

Hemelrijk, C. K., & Hildenbrandt, H. (2012). Schools of fish and flocks of birds: Their shape and internal structure by self-organization. *Interface Focus, 2*(6), 726–737.

Hinton, G. E. (1989). Learning distributed representations of concepts. In R. G. M. Morris (Ed.), *Parallel distributed processing: Implications for psychology and neurobiology* (pp. 46–61). Clarendon Press.

Hiratani, N., & Fukai, T. (2015). Signal variability reduction and prior expectation generation through wiring plasticity. *bioRxiv.* https://doi.org/10.1101/024406

Hocevar, D. (1980). Intelligence, divergent thinking, and creativity. *Intelligence, 4*(1), 25–40.

Hohwy, J. (2007). The sense of self in the phenomenology of agency and perception. *Psyche, 13*(1), 1–20.

Hommel, B. (2001). The theory of event coding (TEC): A framework for perception and action planning. *Behavioral and Brain Sciences, 24*(5), 849–878.

Hurford, J. R. (2003). The neural basis of predicate-argument structure. *Behavioral and Brain Sciences, 26*(3), 261–283.

Husserl, E. (1970). *Logical investigations* (2nd ed.) (J. N. Findlay, Trans.). Routledge. (Original work published 1913, 1921)

Husserl, E. (1993). *Early writings in the philosophy of logic and mathematics* (D. Willard, Trans.). Kluwer. (Original work published 1890–1908).

Johnson, M., & Lakoff, G. (2002). Why cognitive linguistics requires embodied realism. *Cognitive Linguistics, 13*(3), 245–264.

Kempson, R. M. (Ed.). (1988). *Mental representations: The interface between language and reality.* Cambridge University Press.

Koestler, A. (1964). *The act of creation.* Hutchinson.

Kühn, S., Haggard, P., & Brass, M. (2009). Intentional inhibition: How the 'veto-area' exerts control. *Human Brain Mapping, 30*(9), 2834–2843.

Lakoff, G. (2012). Explaining embodied cognition results. *Topics in Cognitive Science, 4*(4), 773–785.

Leiner, B. M., Cerf, V. G., Clark, D. D., Kahn, R. E., Kleinrock, L., Lynch, D. C., Postel, J., Roberts, L. G., & Wolff, S. (1997). *Brief history of internet.* Internet Society.

Lenneberg, E. H. (1967). *The biological foundations of language.* Wiley.

Lewis, M. D. (2002). The dialogical brain: Contributions of emotional neurobiology to understanding the dialogical self. *Theory & Psychology, 12*(2), 175–190.

Little, D. Y., & Sommer, F. T. (2011). Learning in embodied action-perception loops through exploration. *arXiv,* 1112–1125.

Little, D. Y., & Sommer, F. T. (2013). Learning and exploration in action-perception loops. *Frontiers in Neural Circuits, 7,* 37.

MacDonald, C., & MacDonald, G. (Eds.). (1995). *Connectionism: Debates on psychological explanation.* Blackwell.

Macquarrie, J. (1972). *Existentialism.* Westminster.

Malenka, R. C., & Bear, M. F. (2004). LTP and LTD: An embarrassment of riches. *Neuron, 44* (1), 5–21.

Martin, M. G. F. (1995). Bodily awareness: A sense of ownership. In J. L. Bermúdez, A. J. Marcel, & N. Eilan (Eds.), *The body and the self* (pp. 267–289). MIT Press.

Merleau-Ponty, M. (1992). The nature of perception (F. William, Trans.). In H. J. Silverman & J. Barry (Eds.), *Text and dialogues* (pp. 74–84). Humanities Press. (Original work published 1933)

Mill, J. S. (1893). *A system of logic, ratiocinative and inductive: Being a connected view of the principles of evidence and the methods of scientific investigation.* Longmans, green, and Company.

Miller, R. (1991). *Cortico-hippocampal interplay and the representation of contexts in the brain.* Springer Science & Business Media.

Mitchell, R. W. (1993). Mental models of mirror-self-recognition: Two theories. *New Ideas in Psychology, 11*, 295–325.

Morris, D. J. (1978). *Manwatching: A field guide to human behaviour.* Abrams.

Northoff, G., Heinzel, A., De Greck, M., Bermpohl, F., Dobrowolny, H., & Panksepp, J. (2006). Self-referential processing in our brain—A meta-analysis of imaging studies on the self. *Neuroimage, 31*(1), 440–457.

O'Brien, E. J., Rizzella, M. L., Albrecht, J. E., & Halleran, J. G. (1998). Updating a situation model: A memory-based text processing view. *Journal of Experimental Psychology: Learning, Memory, and Cognition, 24*(5), 1200.

Paller, K. A., & Voss, J. L. (2004). Memory reactivation and consolidation during sleep. *Learning & Memory, 11*, 664–670.

Pavlov, D. S., & Kasumyan, A. O. (2000). Patterns and mechanisms of schooling behavior in fish: A review. *Journal of Ichthyology, 40*(2), 163.

Piaget, J., & Inhelder, B. (1969). *The psychology of the child* (H. Weaver, Trans.). Basic Books.

Pinker, S. (1994). *The language instinct: The new science of language and mind.* Penguin.

Prinz, W. (1997). Perception and action planning. *European Journal of Cognitive Psychology, 9*, 129–154.

Pryzwara, E. (2014). *Analogia entis: Metaphysics: original structure and universal rhythm* (J. R. Betz & D. B. Hart, Trans.). Eerdmans.

Rizzolatti, G., Fadiga, L., Gallese, V., & Fogassi, L. (1996). Premotor cortex and the recognition of motor actions. *Cognitive Brain Research, 3*, 131–141.

Roese, N. J. (1994). The functional basis of counterfactual thinking. *Journal of Personality and Social Psychology, 66*(5), 805.

Rolls, E. T. (1989). Parallel distributed processing in the brain: Implication of the functional architecture of neuronal networks in the hippocampus. In R. G. M. Morris (Ed.), *Parallel distributed processing: Implications for psychology and neurobiology* (pp. 286–308). Clarendon Press.

Rovee-Collier, C. (1995). Time windows in cognitive development. *Developmental Psychology, 31*(2), 147–169.

Rumelhart, D. E., McClelland, J. L., & PDP Research Group. (1987a). *Parallel distributed processing.* MIT Press.

Rumelhart, D. E., Smolensky, P., McClelland, J. L., & Hinton, G. E. (1987b). Schemata and sequential thought processes in PDP models. In D. E. Rumelhart, J. L. McClelland, & PDP Research Group (Eds.), *Parallel distributed processing* (pp. 7–57). MIT Press.

Slabakova, R. (2006). Is there a critical period for semantics? *Second Language Research, 22*(3), 302–338.

Schacter, D. L., Addis, D. R., & Buckner, R. L. (2007). Remembering the past to imagine the future: The prospective brain. *Nature Reviews Neuroscience, 8*(9), 657.

Schneider, F., Bermpohl, F., Heinzel, A., Rotte, M., Walter, M., Tempelmann, C., Wiebking, C., Dobrowolny, H., Heinze, H. J., & Northoff, G. (2008). The resting brain and our self:

Self-relatedness modulates resting state neural activity in cortical midline structures. *Neuroscience, 157*(1), 120–131.

Schwenkler, J. L. (2008). Mental vs. embodied models of mirrored self-recognition: Some preliminary considerations. In B. Hardy Valee & N. Payette (Eds.), *Beyond the brain: Embodied, situated, and distributed cognition* (pp. 93–105). Cambridge Scholars Press.

Smith, K. S., Berridge, K. C., & Aldridge, J. W. (2011). Disentangling pleasure from incentive salience and learning signals in brain reward circuitry. *Proceedings of the National Academy of Sciences, 108*(27), E255–E264.

Smolensky, P. (1995). Reply: Constituent structure and explanation in an integrated connectionist/symbolic cognitive architecture. In C. MacDonald, & G. MacDonald (Eds.), *Connectionism: Debates on psychological explanation* (Vol. 2, pp. 223–290). Blackwell.

Solé, R. V., Corominas-Murtra, B., Valverde, S., & Steels, L. (2010). Language networks: Their structure, function, and evolution. *Complexity, 15*(6), 20–26.

Sommer, M. A., & Wurtz, R. H. (2008). Brain circuits for the internal monitoring of movements. *Annual Review of Neuroscience, 31*, 317–338.

Squire, L. R. (1987). *Memory and brain.* Oxford University Press.

Stein, E. (1970). *On the problem of empathy* (W. Stein, Trans.). ICS Publications. (Original work published 1916)

Stein, E. (1998). *Potency and act: Studies toward a philosophy of being* (W. Redmond, Trans.). ICS Publications. (Original work published 1931)

Steinberg, L. (2005). Cognitive and affective development in adolescence. *Trends in Cognitive Sciences, 9*(2), 69–74.

Stickgold, R. (1998). Sleep: Off-line memory reprocessing. *Trends in Cognitive Sciences, 2*(12), 484–492.

Stickgold, R. (2005). Sleep-dependent memory consolidation. *Nature, 437*(7063), 1272.

Suls, J. (1983). Cognitive processes in humor appreciation. In P. E. McGhee & J. H. Goldstein (Eds.), *Handbook of humor research* (pp. 39–57). Springer.

Swenson, R., & Turvey, M. T. (1991). Thermodynamic reasons for perception-action cycles. *Ecological Psychology, 3*(4), 317–348.

Synofzik, M., Thier, P., Leube, D. T., Schlotterbeck, P., & Lindner, A. (2009). Misattributions of agency in schizophrenia are based on imprecise predictions about the sensory consequences of one's actions. *Brain, 133*(1), 262–271.

Tomasello, M., & Call, J. (1997). *Primate cognition.* Oxford University Press.

Tomasello, M., Carpenter, M., Call, J., Behne, T., & Moll, H. (2005). Understanding and sharing intentions: The origins of cultural cognition. *Behavioral and Brain Sciences, 28*(5), 675–735.

Tulving, E. (1985). *Elements of episodic memory.* Oxford Science Publications.

Turvey, M. T., & Fitzpatrick, P. (1993). Commentary: Development of perception-action systems and general principles of pattern formation. *Child Development, 64*(4), 1175–1190.

Twenge, J. M. (2017). *IGen: Why today's super-connected kids are growing up less rebellious, more tolerant, less happy—and completely unprepared for adulthood—and what that means for the rest of us.* Simon and Schuster.

van Buuren, M., Vink, M., & Kahn, R. S. (2012). Default-mode network dysfunction and self-referential processing in healthy siblings of schizophrenia patients. *Schizophrenia Research, 142*(1), 237–243.

Vogeley, K., & Fink, G. R. (2003). Neural correlates of the first-person-perspective. *Trends in Cognitive Sciences, 7*(1), 38–42.

Wamsley, E. J. (2014). Dreaming and offline memory consolidation. *Current Neurology and Neuroscience Reports, 14*(3), 433.

Wamsley, E. J., & Stickgold, R. (2010). Dreaming and offline memory processing. *Current Biology, 20*(23), R1010–R1013.

Wiedemann, C. (2007). Memory consolidation . . . while you are sleeping. *Nature Reviews Neuroscience, 8*(2), 86–88.

Wisniewski, E. J. (1997). When concepts combine. *Psychonomic Bulletin & Review, 4*(2), 167–183.

Yu, C. T. (1988). *Being and relation: A theological critique of western dualism and individualism (theology and science at the frontiers of knowledge).* Scottish Academic Press.

Zwaan, R. A., & Radvansky, G. A. (1998). Situation models in language comprehension and memory. *Psychological Bulletin, 123*(2), 162.

7. Representation Failure and Psychopathology

Amit, D. (1989). *Modeling brain function: The world of attractor neural networks.* Cambridge University Press.

Chen, E. Y. H. (1994). A neural network model of cortical information processing in schizophrenia. I: Interaction between biological and social factors in symptom formation. *The Canadian Journal of Psychiatry, 39*(8), 362–367.

Chen, E. Y. H. (1995). A neural network model of cortical information processing in schizophrenia. II: Role of hippocampal-cortical interaction: A review and a model. *The Canadian Journal of Psychiatry, 40*(1), 21–26.

Crow, T. J. (1980). Molecular pathology of schizophrenia: More than one disease process? *British Journal of Medical Psychology, 280,* 66–68.

Crow, T. J. (1982). Two syndromes in schizophrenia? *Trends in Neurosciences, 5,* 351–354.

Eichenbaum, H., Schoenbaum, G., Young, B., & Bunsey, M. (1996). Functional organization of the hippocampal memory system. *Proceedings of the National Academy of Sciences of the USA, 93*(24), 13500–13507.

Hoffman, R. E., & McGlashan, T. H. (1993). Parallel distributed processing and the emergence of schizophrenic symptoms. *Schizophrenia Bulletin, 19*(1), 119–140.

Jackson, J. H. (1932). *Selected writings of John Hughlings Jackson* (J. Taylor, Ed.). Hodder and Stoughton.

Jaspers, K. (1963). *General psychopathology* (J. Hoenig & M. W. Hamilton, Trans.). Manchester University Press. (Original work published 1913)

Keysar, B., Lin, S., & Barr, D. J. (2003). Limits on theory of mind use in adults. *Cognition, 89*(1), 25–41.

Miller, R. (2008). *A neurodynamic theory of schizophrenia and related disorders.* Lulu Press.

Phillips, W. A., & Silverstein, S. M. (2003). Convergence of biological and psychological perspectives on cognitive coordination in schizophrenia. *Behavioral and Brain Sciences, 26*(1), 65–82.

Rolls, E. T. (1996). A theory of hippocampal function in memory. *Hippocampus, 6*(6), 601–620.

Rumelhart, D. E., McClelland, J. L., & PDP Research Group. (1987). *Parallel distributed processing.* MIT Press.

Serrano-Pedraza, I., Romero-Ferreiro, V., Read, J. C., Diéguez-Risco, T., Bagney, A., Caballero-González, M., Rodríguez-Torresano, J., & Rodriguez-Jimenez, R. (2014). Reduced visual surround suppression in schizophrenia shown by measuring contrast detection thresholds. *Frontiers in Psychology, 5,* 1431.

Sherman, J. W., Macrae, C. N., & Bodenhausen, G. V. (2011). Attention and Stereotyping: Cognitive constraints on the construction of meaningful social impressions. *European Review of Social Psychology, 11*(1), 145–175.

Silverstein, S. M., & Keane, B. P. (2011). Perceptual organization impairment in schizophrenia and associated brain mechanisms: Review of research from 2005 to 2010. *Schizophrenia Bulletin, 37*(4), 690–699.

Singer, W. (2000). Phenomenal awareness and consciousness from a neurobiological perspective. *Neural Correlates of Consciousness: Empirical and Conceptual Questions,* 121–137.

Smolensky, P. (1995). Reply: Constituent structure and explanation in an integrated connectionist/symbolic cognitive architecture. In C. MacDonald & G. MacDonald (Eds.), *Connectionism: Debates on psychological explanation* (Vol. 2, pp. 223–290). Blackwell.

Thom, R. (1975). *Structural stability and morphogenesis: An outline of a general theory of models* (D. H. Fowler, Trans.). W. A. Benjamin. (Original work published 1972)

Uhlhaas, P. J., & Singer, W. (2010). Abnormal neural oscillations and synchrony in schizophrenia. *Nature Reviews Neuroscience, 11*(2), 100.

Zeeman, C. (1977). *Catastrophe theory: Selected papers 1972–1977.* Addison-Wesley.

8. Towards a New Representational Framework in Psychopathology

Andreasen, N. C. (1979). Thought, language, and communication disorders: II. Diagnostic significance. *Archives of General Psychiatry, 36*(12), 1325–1330.

Arnett, J. J. (2000). Emerging adulthood: A theory of development from the late teens through the twenties. *American Psychologist, 55*(5), 469–480.

Baron-Cohen, S., Leslie, A. M., & Frith, U. (1985). Does the autistic child have a 'theory of mind'? *Cognition, 21*(1), 37–46.

Blackmore, S. (1999). *The meme machine.* Oxford University Press.

Borsboom, D. (2017). A network theory of mental disorders. *World Psychiatry, 16*(1), 5–13.

Chaika, E. (1995). On analyzing schizophrenic speech: What model should we use? *Speech and Language Disorders in Psychiatry* (pp. 47–56). Gaskell.

Dawkins, R. (1976). *The selfish gene.* Oxford University Press.

Fauconnier, G., & Turner, M. (2008). *The way we think: Conceptual blending and the mind's hidden complexities.* Basic Books.

Feinberg, T. E., Schindler, R. J., Flanagan, N. G., & Haber, L. D. (1992). Two alien hand syndromes. *Neurology, 42*(1), 19.

Fish, F. J., & Hamilton, M. (1985). *Fish's clinical psychopathology: Signs and symptoms in psychiatry* (2nd ed). Wright.

Frau, R., Orrù, M., Puligheddu, M., Gessa, G. L., Mereu, G., Marrosu, F., & Bortolato, M. (2008). Sleep deprivation disrupts prepulse inhibition of the startle reflex: Reversal by antipsychotic drugs. *Internal Journal of Neuropsychopharmacology, 11,* 947–955.

Frith, C. D. (2004). Schizophrenia and theory of mind. *Psychological Medicine, 34*(3), 385–389.

Frith, C. D., & Done, D. J. (1989). Experiences of alien control in schizophrenia reflect a disorder in the central monitoring of action. *Psychological Medicine, 19*(2), 359–363.

Frith, C. D., & Corcoran, R. (1996). Exploring 'theory of mind' in people with schizophrenia. *Psychological Medicine, 26*(3), 521–530.

Goldberg, G. (1985). Supplementary motor area structure and function: Review and hypotheses. *Behavioral and Brain Sciences, 8*(4), 567–588.

Graesser, A. C., Bowers, C., Olde, B., & Pomeroy, V. (1999). Who said what? Source memory for narrator and character agents in literary short stories. *Journal of Educational Psychology, 91*(2), 284.

Green, M. J., & Philips, M. L. (2004). Social threat perception and the evolution of paranoia. *Neuroscience and Biobehavioral Reviews, 28*, 333–342.

Grundlingh, L. (2017). Memes as speech acts. *Social Semiotics, 28*(2), 147–168.

Harpending, H., & Cochran, G. (2009). *The 10,000-year explosion.* Basic Books.

Haselton, M.G., Nettle, D., & Murray, D. R. (2015). The evolution of cognitive bias. In D. M. Buss (Ed.), *The handbook of evolutionary psychology* (2nd ed., Vol. 2, pp. 968–987). Wiley.

Hensch, T. K. (2005). Critical period plasticity in local cortical circuits. *Nature Reviews Neuroscience, 6*(11), 877–888.

Hermans, H. J. M., & Kempen, H. J. G. (1993). *The dialogical self: meaning as movement.* Academic Press.

Hermans, H. J. M., & Dimaggio, G. (2007). Self, identity, and globalization in times of uncertainty: A dialogical analysis. *Review of General Psychology, 11*(1), 31.

Humphrey, N. (1986). *The inner eye.* Faber and Faber.

Jaspers, K. (1963). *General psychopathology* (J. Hoenig & M. W. Hamilton, Trans.). Manchester University Press. (Original work published 1913)

Jones, S. R., & Fernyhough, C. (2007). Neural correlates of inner speech and auditory verbal hallucinations: A critical review and theoretical integration. *Clinical Psychology Review, 27*(2), 140–154.

Lewis, M. D. (2002). The dialogical brain: Contributions of emotional neurobiology to understanding the dialogical self. *Theory & Psychology, 12*(2), 175–190.

Lhermitte, F. (1986). Human autonomy and the frontal lobes. Part II: Patient behavior in complex and social situations: The 'environmental dependency syndrome'. *Annals of Neurology, 19*(4), 335–343.

Longenecker, J., Hui, C., Chen, E. Y. H., & Elvevag, B. (2016). Concepts of 'self' in delusion resolution. *Schizophrenia Research Cognition, 3*, 8–10.

Lorenz, K. (1981). *The foundations of ethology* (K. Lorenz & R. W. Kickert, Trans.). Springer-Verlag.

McGlashan, T. H., & Hoffman, R. E. (2000). Schizophrenia as a disorder of developmentally reduced synaptic connectivity. *Archives of General Psychiatry, 57*, 637–648.

McGuire, P. K., David, A. S., Murray, R. M., Frackowiak, R. S. J., Frith, C. D., Wright, I., & Silbersweig, D. A. (1995). Abnormal monitoring of inner speech: A physiological basis for auditory hallucinations. *The Lancet, 346*(8975), 596–600.

McGuire, P. K., Silbersweig, D. A., Wright, I., Murray, R. M., Frackowiak, R. S., & Frith, C. D. (1996). The neural correlates of inner speech and auditory verbal imagery in schizophrenia: Relationship to auditory verbal hallucinations. *British Journal of Psychiatry, 169*(2), 148–159.

McKenna, P. J., & Oh, T. M. (2005). *Schizophrenic speech: Making sense of bathroots and ponds that fall in doorways.* Cambridge University Press.

Moscovitch, M. (1995). Confabulation. In D. L. Schacter, J. T. Coyle, G. D. Fischbach, M. M. Mesulum, & L. G. Sullivan (Eds.), *Memory distortion* (pp. 226–251). Harvard University Press.

Petrovsky, N., Ettinger, U., Hill, A., Frenzel, L., Meyhofer, I., Wagner, M., Backhaus, J., & Kumari, V. (2014). Sleep deprivation disrupts prepulse inhibition and induces psychosis-like symptoms in healthy humans. *Journal of Neuroscience, 34*(27), 9134–9140.

Piaget, J., & Inhelder, B. (1969). *The psychology of the child* (H. Weaver, Trans.). Basic Books.

Samuels, A. (1985). *Jung and the post-Jungians.* Routledge & Kegan Paul.

Scheneider, K. (1959). *Clinical psychopathology.* Grune and Stratton.

Senkfor, A. J., & Van Petten, C. (1998). Who said what? An event-related potential investigation of source and item memory. *Journal of Experimental Psychology: Learning, Memory, and Cognition, 24*(4), 1005.

Sims, A. (Ed.). (1995). *Speech and language disorders in psychiatry: Proceedings of the Fifth Leeds Psychopathology Symposium* (Vol. 5). American Psychiatric Publishing.

Stein, D. J., & Ludik, J. (Eds.). (1998). *Neural networks and psychopathology: Connectionist models in practice and research.* Cambridge University Press.

Tulving, E. (1972). Episodic and semantic memory. In E. Tulving & W. Donaldson (Eds.), *Organization of memory* (pp. 382–402). Academic Press.

Wernicke, C. (2005). *An outline of psychiatry in clinical lectures: The lectures of Carl Wernicke* (R. Miller, & J. Dennison, Eds.). Springer. (Original work published 1881).

9. Psychopathological Evaluation: The Clinical Dialogue

Argyle, M. (1975). *Bodily communication.* Methuen.

Chen, E. Y. H., Lam, L. C., Kan, C. S., Chan, C. K., Kwok, C. L., Nguyen, D. G. H., & Chen, R. Y. (1996). Language disorganisation in schizophrenia: Validation and assessment with a new clinical rating instrument. *Hong Kong Journal of Psychiatry, 6*(1), 4–13.

Elstein, A. S., & Schwarz, A. (2002). Clinical problem solving and diagnostic decision making: Selective review of the cognitive literature. *British Medical Journal, 324*(7339), 729–732.

Garrod, S., & Pickering, M. J. (2009). Joint action, interactive alignment, and dialogue. *Topics in Cognitive Science, 1*(2), 292–304.

Geertz, C. (1973). *The interpretation of cultures: Selected essays.* Basic Books.

Good, B. (1993). *Medicine, rationality, and experience.* Cambridge University Press.

Grice, H. P. (1975). Logic and conversation. In P. Cole & J. L. Morgan (Eds.), *Syntax and semantics 3: Speech acts* (pp. 41–58). Academic Press.

Husserl, E. (1931). *Ideas: General introduction to pure phenomenology* (W. R. B. Gibson, Trans.). Macmillan. (Original work published 1913)

Husserl, E. (1954). *The crisis of the European sciences and transcendental phenomenology: An introduction to phenomenological philosophy* (D. Carr, Trans.). Northwestern University Press. (Original work published 1936)

Husserl, E. (1970). *Logical investigations* (2nd ed.) (J. N. Findlay, Trans.). Routledge. (Original work published 1913, 1921)

Iser, W. (1978). *The act of reading: A theory of aesthetic response.* The Johns Hopkins University Press.

Jaspers, K. (1963). *General psychopathology* (J. Hoenig & M. W. Hamilton, Trans.). Manchester University Press. (Original work published 1913)

Libby, L. K., Shaeffer, E. M., & Eibach, R. P. (2009). Seeing meaning in action: A bidirectional link between visual perspective and action identification level. *Journal of Experimental Psychology: General, 138*(4), 503.

Marková, I. (2005). *Insight in psychiatry*. Cambridge University Press.

Neisser, U. (1989). From direct perception to conceptual structure. In *Concepts and conceptual development: Ecological and intellectual factors in categorization* (pp. 11–24). CUP Archive.

Nimmon, L., & Stenfors-Hayes, T. (2016). The 'handling' of power in the physician-patient encounter: Perceptions from experienced physicians. *BMC Medical Education, 16*(1), 53–73.

Oswald, D., Sherratt, F., & Smith, S. (2014). Handling the Hawthorne effect: The challenges surrounding a participant observer. *Review of Social Studies, 1*(1), 53–73.

Pickering, M. J., & Garrod, S. (2004). Toward a mechanistic psychology of dialogue. *Behavioral and Brain Sciences, 27*(2), 169–190.

Ricoeur, P. (1981). *Hermeneutics and the human sciences: Essays on language, action and Interpretation* (J. B. Thompson, Ed.). Cambridge University Press.

Robins, R. W., Spranca, M. D., & Mendelsohn, G. A. (1996). The actor-observer effect revisited: Effects of individual differences and repeated social interactions on actor and observer attributions. *Journal of Personality and Social Psychology, 71*(2), 375–389.

Roter, D. L., & Hall, J. A. (2006). *Doctors talking with patients/patients talking with doctors: Improving communication in medical visits* (2nd ed.). Praeger.

Russell, J. A. (1991). Culture and the categorization of emotions. *Psychological Bulletin, 110*(3), 426–450.

Shea, S. C. (1998). *Psychiatric interviewing: The art of understanding: A practical guide for psychiatrists, psychologists, nurses and other health professionals* (2nd ed.). W. B. Saunders.

Tait, L., Birchwood, M., & Trower, P. (2003). Predicting engagement with services for psychosis: Insight, symptoms and recovery style. *British Journal of Psychiatry, 182*(2), 123–128.

Zwaan, R. A., & Radvansky, G. A. (1998). Situation models in language comprehension and memory. *Psychological Bulletin, 123*(2), 162–185.

Index

accommodation. *See also* assimilation; as in cognitive development, 76, 145, 190

action-perception models, 82–83, 102, 108, 113; perception-action model, 69

activation, weighted, 31. *See also* neurocomputational model

actualization, 50, 58–59

acute confusional state, 130

addressing, as in idea of reference, 133, 138, 156

adolescence, 81, 153–55

aesthetic experiences, 48–49, 65

affective network, 131. *See also* neurocomputational model

agency, sense of, 62, 67, 95, 134–36, 144, 156; in digitalisation, 100

alien hand syndrome, 136

alignment. *See under* clinical dialogue

animal guessing game, 166

animated object, 63, 77. *See also* object: empirically external

anorexia nervosa, 96

AP cycle (action-perception cycle). *See* action-perception models

archetypes, 142

assimilation. *See also* accommodation; as in cognitive development, 76

atomic unit of experience, 52–53

attention, joint, as in self development, 94, 114

attention, shared. *See* attention, joint, as in self development

auditory scene analysis, 92, 181

authenticity, 48, 59–60, 190

autism, 140–42, 152

auto-associative network, 32 fig. 2.5, 104, 108 fig. 6.12

autobiographical information. *See under* information

auto-contact behaviour, 113

automaticity, 130, 156. *See also* Bakhtinization

back-engineering process, 92

Bakhtinization, 136, 139–41. *See also* automaticity

becoming, process of, 53

Berrios, German Elias, 1–2

Bias Against Disconfirmatory Evidence, 90

bi-association, 113

bipolar disorders, 154

bizarre representation. *See under* mental representation

borderline personality disorder, 132

bottom-up processes, 168

brain markers, 7–8

brain, as an 'information-consuming' organ, 16

carbohydrates, preference for, 37

catastrophe theory, 121–23

choice, 61–63, 68, 106–7, 114, 130, 153–54, 172; freedom of, 62, 79; in digitalisation, 100; individual, 79 fig. 5.5, 154; passive, 62

circumstantial speech, 149, 151